Interpersonal Communication in Nursing

For Churchill Livingstone

Commissioning Editor: Ellen Green
Project Development Editor: Mairi McCubbin
Design Direction: Judith Wright
Project Manager: Valerie Burgess
Project Controller: Pat Miller
Production Desktop Unit: Neil Dickson
Pre-press Desktop Operator: Kate Walshaw
Sales Promotion Executive: Hilary Brown

Interpersonal Communication in Nursing

Theory and Practice

Edited by

Roger B. Ellis BSc CertEd MEd DipStudCouns
Independent counsellor and trainer, Lincoln

Robert J. Gates BEd(Hons) MSc CertEd RMN RNMH DipNurs(Lond) RNT
Lecturer in Nursing, University of Hull.
Head of Profession – Learning Disability Nursing, Hull and Holderness NHS Community Trust

Neil Kenworthy MBA BEd RGN RMN
Management and Education Consultant, PNK Associates, Lincoln

CHURCHILL LIVINGSTONE
EDINBURGH HONG KONG LONDON MADRID MELBOURNE NEW YORK AND TOKYO 1995

CHURCHILL LIVINGSTONE
Medical Division of Pearson Professional Limited

Distributed in the United States of America by Churchill
Livingstone, 650 Avenue of the Americas, New York,
N.Y. 10011, and by associated companies, branches and
representatives throughout the world.

© Pearson Professional Limited 1995

First published 1995

ISBN 0 443 04996 3

British Library Cataloguing in Publication Data
A catalogue record for this book is available from
the British Library.

Library of Congress Cataloging in Publication Data
A catalog record for this book is available from
the Library of Congress.

The
publisher's
policy is to use
**paper manufactured
from sustainable forests**

Printed in Singapore

Contents

Contributors

Andrew M. Betts MEd RMN AdvDipCouns CPNCert CertEd
Specialist Subject Leader, Mid-Trent College of Nursing and Midwifery, Lincoln
5 Improving communication
9 The counselling relationship

Tepi Corbett (Terttu Marsatta) BA RGN DipN CertEd RNT
Part-time lecturer in Nursing Studies, University of Hull
7 A nurse's work relationships

Patricia East BEd(Hons) CertEd MA DipStudCouns AdvCertPsychotherapy
Independent counsellor and psychotherapist, Lincoln
8 The mentoring relationship

Roger B. Ellis BSc CertEd MEd DipStudCouns
Independent counsellor and trainer, Lincoln
1 Defining communication
2 The person in communication

Robert J. Gates MSc BEd(Hons) RMN RMNH DipN(Lond) RNT CertEd
Lecturer in Nursing, University of Hull, Head of Profession-Learning Disability Nursing, Hull and Holderness NHS Community Trust
2 The person in communication
6 Communicating in groups

Stuart A. Hindle BSc(Hons) RGN RMN RNT CertEd
Nurse Teacher, Bede, Newcastle and Northumbria College of Health Studies, Freeman Hospital, Newcastle-upon-Tyne
4 Psychological factors affecting communication

Peter A. Morrall MSc BA(Hons) CertEd RGN RMN RMNH
Principal Lecturer in Nursing Studies/Sociology of Health and Illness, and Section Leader, Nursing Studies, School of Human Studies, University of Teesside, Middlesborough
3 Social factors affecting communication

Preface

This book is primarily for students undertaking diploma programmes that lead to a first-level nursing and midwifery qualification. Registered nurses and midwives taking post-registration courses may also find it useful.

Radical changes in nurse education, through Project 2000, have resulted in a need for a book that covers the theory and practice of communication in sufficient depth to meet the rigorous academic demands of diploma programmes. This book provides a sound basic grounding in the fundamental concepts, principles and ideas, and the different theoretical perspectives of communication. It then uses these to illuminate typical interactions in the daily life of the professional carer. Practical applications from nursing are used to support the theory, throughout the book.

The focus of the book is on enabling students to make sense of the face-to-face communication they experience by actively reflecting on it. The theoretical ideas do not stand alone, but support this central activity of becoming more objective and analytical about personal ways of communicating, which often go unnoticed or are taken for granted. By challenging them to examine encounters with others from a variety of perspectives, the authors hope that student communication will become more intentional and effective.

The contents of the book fit into three sections. The first two chapters consider communication and the person; what it is, and why and how individuals communicate. The second section looks at factors affecting communication and how it may be improved, and at the dynamics of the group setting. In the final section of the book the use of communication in establishing and developing relationships is examined, at an interpersonal level.

The editors believe that the advantages of this book are that it:

- is specifically applied to nurses and nursing
- satisfies the needs of students who require a breadth of information
- focuses on the real world of students and their communication needs
- offers a range of alternative models
- provides practical assignments set in differing nursing contexts.

As nurses gain insight into the complexities of communication they realise its importance not only for interpersonal relationships in general, but in ensuring the quality and success of patient care and treatment.

R. E.
B. G.
Lincoln 1994   N. K.

Acknowledgement

The editors wish to give special thanks to Andy Betts who has given generous personal and professional support from the early days of the preparation of this book.

Emphasis on theory

1

Defining communication

Roger Ellis

DEFINING COMMUNICATION

Human beings have a built-in drive to relate to each other. A baby's very survival depends on getting its caretaker to attend to its needs. The effectiveness and happiness of adults is directly linked to a capacity to form satisfying relationships. The stability and health of any organisation depend on dealing successfully with the complexity of its internal relationships and having effective ways of relating to the outside world. The same applies to nations and countries on the international political scene.

When relationships break down or become a source of stress the central complaint is commonly that of poor communication. 'I just can't get through to my boss. She doesn't seem to want to know what I'm saying'. Often problems in relating stem from the process of communication itself rather than what is being communicated. 'It's not so much *what* he said but the way he said it that irritated me so much'.

Appeal to common experience bears out these generalisations. Most people have felt anger and helplessness at not being listened to when saying something important. Also, the intense frustration of being misunderstood when the other person refuses or does not take the trouble to see things from your point of view. Equally, it is disturbing to realise that someone is saying one thing but meaning another. This is true not only in intimate relationships in personal life but also at work where the focus is on a job that has to be done.

These comments apply to people interacting with each other—the interpersonal world. There is also another world of communication within each person, the intra-psychic world. Comments such as 'He's his own worst enemy' or 'She's so critical of herself' suggest that reference to this internal communication is necessary to do justice to the rich complexity of human experience. It seems that people live simultaneously in the outside world and in an internal world of thought and feeling. For some personalities the inter-personal world is the most rewarding and is where they focus their attention. For others the intra-psychic world is the most real and offers the greatest rewards. Perhaps we are all seeking a balance between the two.

What is true about relations and communications between individuals and groups is also true about the internal thoughts and feelings of every human being. If the need to communicate with and explore other people is so strong why do so many people find it difficult and un-rewarding? For some, relating to other people is considered risky or even dangerous and therefore the need for safety and security dominates the need to relate. Langs (1983) puts it thus:

> Communicative exchanges give substance to our lives; they are essential for survival and growth. We know that we require a sufficient amount of internal communication, as in private thoughts, fantasies and dreams to maintain our sanity. The need for expression is powerful in all human beings, although often it is compromised by strong needs for defence, non-communication, and withdrawal. Self-expression is important to all coping efforts and especially so in emotionally trying situations.

THE FOCUS OF THIS BOOK

Of all the ways of expressing thoughts and feelings—a political address, a dream, intimate words of affection, a poem or play, a scientific report, a painting, a piece of music—the focus of this book is on communication between individuals using the spoken word and associated elements. The communication can be between two individuals or a group of people and is assumed to be in a professional nursing setting, for example, nurse/patient, nurse/nurse or nurse/doctor/manager.

This apparently simple process of one person talking to another is highly complex and subtle and needs to be analysed carefully if it is to be understood. Chapter 1 attempts to do this by defining the basic components of communication, outlining a specific model of communication and by building a fuller picture bit by bit to do justice to the complexity. Later chapters examine the influences which affect communication and how communication might be improved, as well as looking at communication in various settings.

THE BASIC COMPONENTS OF COMMUNICATION

SENDER, MESSAGE, RECEIVER

The basic unit of communication is made up of a sender, a receiver and a message set within a particular context (Fig. 1.1). The sender intends to convey a particular message but may send much that is beyond direct awareness. The unconscious or hidden content of communication is an integral and important part of the whole. The message itself may be in line with conscious intentions or may be at considerable variance with them. Equally the receiver may register what was intended to be sent but often receives more as well, especially the unconscious component. The four variables interact, each contributing to the meaning of a communication.

In the example given in Box 1.1, the community psychiatric nurse might perceive how depressed the patient is in contradiction of the explicit message. A more naive observer might not pick up this message at all.

This simple diagram models a one-way communication only. Some people act as though there is no response to what they are communicating

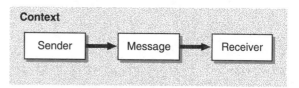

Figure 1.1   The basic components of communication

Box 1.1	The basic components of communication: example

Sender: patient
Message: I'm feeling just fine today
Receiver: community psychiatric nurse
Context: home visit

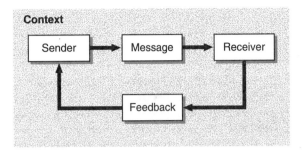

Figure 1.2 Basic components of communication with feedback

but the focus here is on two-way communication where the receiver is actively involved in the process so that each person is modifying messages in the light of the other's response. Nevertheless, one-way communication is common even in the face-to-face situation between a doctor/nurse and nurse/patient. 'You should have been aware of the problems of this patient much sooner, nurse'. 'You're not to have anything to eat for 24 hours'.

Many who assent to two-way communication in theory do not practise it. Bradley & Edinberg (1990) give the following reasons why nurses may use one-way communication though they believe in a two-way model:

• The communicator controls one-way communication. Clearly, listening to a response makes demands on the nurse's capacity to adapt to the unexpected and she may feel more vulnerable or intimate with the patient as a result.
• One-way communication can take place more easily whilst doing something else, e.g. whilst making the bed. Full attention on the receiver is not always necessary.
• Nurses feel under pressure to do lots of tasks. Two-way communication may take time away from other important aspects of patient care.

Menzies-Lyth (1960) studied the ways in which the social system of a hospital was organised to protect staff from being overwhelmed by the stress and anxiety generated by their jobs. Amongst these she noted the splitting up of the nurse/patient relationship by breaking down the total workload of a ward into lists of tasks each of which is allocated to a particular nurse. As a result the nurse has restricted contact with any one patient. Another technique she noted was that of depersonalisation, categorisation, and denial of the significance of the individual. These and other devices inhibit the development of a full person-to-person relationship between nurse and patient, with its consequent anxiety.

It is well worth considering other reasons from your own personal experience as to why one-way communication might be adopted and to remain alert to the consequences of one-way and two-way communication in practice.

With a feedback loop the first diagram now becomes a two-way communication (Fig. 1.2).

BASIC PRINCIPLES OF COMMUNICATION

Before developing a more elaborate model it may be helpful to consider four basic principles of communication based on the ideas of Watzlawick et al (1967) summarised in Box 1.2 and described in more detail here.

1. *One cannot **not** communicate.* All behaviour has a message of some sort so that as well as the more obvious carriers of messages like words or gestures, saying or doing nothing is itself a message. Not smiling is just as potent a message as smiling. Once a message has been sent it cannot be retracted. If a judge tells the

Box 1.2	Watzlawick's four basic principles of communication

1. One cannot *not* communicate.
2. Every communication has a content and relationship aspect such that the latter classifies the former and is therefore a metacommunication.
3. A series of communications can be viewed as an uninterrupted series of interchanges.
4. All communication relationships are either symmetrical or complementary depending on whether they are based on equality or inequality.

jury to disregard the evidence given she cannot change the fact that the members have heard it. All communication is irreversible—as many a public figure has learned to her cost.

2. *Every communication has a content and relationship aspect such that the latter classifies the former and is therefore a metacommunication.* Any communication sequence has a message content and also has aspects which refer to the way in which the message is received. How communicators relate to each other is sometimes consciously controlled but is more commonly unconsciously controlled. Consider this exchange:

   Patient: I don't want to take these pills.
   Nurse: You must. Doctor says so.

   The last comment is a communication about the communication (a metacommunication) and marks out clearly how the nurse sees her relationship to the patient—that of control. Chapter 3 looks in more detail at the effects of role and social context on communication.

3. *A series of communications can be viewed as an uninterrupted series of interchanges.* There is no clear beginning or ending to a series of interchanges: any communication between two individuals has a history and a future in itself and is affected by the totality of the past experiences of each individual. Hurtful past experiences can set up a pattern in which the person ignores the offender who then ignores the offended and thus the situation becomes an unhelpful communication chain reaction. It is difficult to deal with this pattern when a patient's manner is habitually offensive.

4. *All communication relationships are either symmetrical or complementary, depending on whether they are based on equality or inequality.* With two equal partners, such as two close friends, the interaction is likely to be symmetrical. With a status or power differential between two people, such as a teacher and pupil or doctor and nurse, the complementary relationship (one 'superior' to the other) will affect any communication between them. In general, how any communication is interpreted depends on the relationship the sender has with the receiver. Again these issues of role, status and power are examined in more detail in Chapter 3.

With four basic principles of communication and a simple model in place it is now possible to develop a more complex model of communication which will form the basis of all further comments in this chapter.

A MODEL OF COMMUNICATION

SENDING A MESSAGE

The model illustrated in Figure 1.3 starts with the thoughts and feelings of the sender i.e. the intrapsychic world, and acknowledges that these have

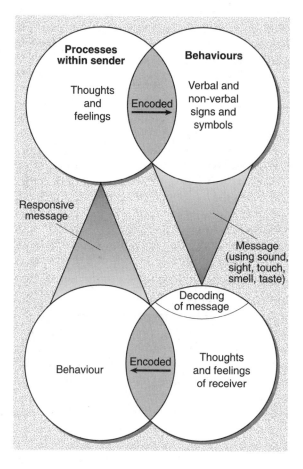

Figure 1.3 A model of communication

to be encoded into some form of behaviour (the message) if they are to leave the internal domain and be communicated to another person (the receiver). The message of verbal and/or non-verbal signs and symbols needs to be carried by one means or another (the channels) on to one or more of the senses of the receiver so that the receiver can perceive it. From this sense data the receiver decodes and interprets the message and has thoughts and feelings as a result. These may or may not match the intended message of the sender. In any interaction the receiver is likely to have thoughts and feelings that she will encode in her own style and send back to the original sender. Thus the process of two-way communication proceeds.

THE MESSAGE

Useful insights into the meaning of a word can often be gained by considering its derivation. The central element in the word 'message' is 'mess' which is still used in two distinct ways—to supply with meals and also to make dirty or untidy with extensions of bungling, interfering, disarranging or man-handling. Hence 'Don't mess with me!'

The derivation of the word message then contains both nurturing qualities and also the potential for confusing and hurting. Messages are indeed sent to create meaning but are also used defensively, to hide what is actually going on, to create confusion and attack relatedness. The work of Laing (1959) and others attempted to demonstrate that a patient's apparently bizarre symptoms (labelled schizophrenic) could make sense if seen in the context of the original patterns of communication in the family which often had the quality of creating confusion and undermining relationships.

Perhaps the most compressed example of the subtlety of the mix of both aspects in a message, nurturing and hurtful, is in the 'double bind' (Bateson et al 1956). The victim of the double bind is caught inside contradictory statements so that she cannot do the right thing. Current pressure in the health service for quality care and for high turnover and efficiency may often be experienced by a nurse as contradictory. One message

received may be clearly incompatible with the next message. Even more difficult to handle is the situation in which the overt message hides or disguises a covert contradictory message. 'Get the turnover rate up' but also implying, but not stating, 'and don't let the quality slip'. The nurse's dilemma is whether to base her action on the overt or the covert message. She is in a double bind, a 'Damned if you do, damned if you don't' situation. Thus messages are often not simple and can appear to be one thing when in fact they are another.

In contrast, the word communicate has no negative overtones, implying only transmitting, making known and passing on of knowledge and information. Related words such as communion and community indicate the emphasis on qualities of sharing and fellowship. Thus communication has the positive and nurturing qualities of message but not the negative, messy ones.

CARRIERS OF THE MESSAGE

In face-to-face communication a message is received through one or more of the five senses. The senses are the means by which a message originating in the external world is registered by the body and converted into internal experience. Messages are conveyed from one person to another through the senses in the following ways.

Language

A highly developed language is the supreme achievement of the human mind and body and is a development beyond the more primitive channels of communication discussed below. Language is necessary for the complex and abstract ideas needed for the intricacies of social organisation and culture. Consider the massive strides forward in civilisation that have taken place since a means was found to express spoken language in written form so that experience and knowledge could last beyond a human lifetime and be transmitted and received other than by face-to-face contact. Consider also the consequences socially and politically of being able to mass produce the written word.

The lexical content of a message, i.e. the words themselves, can only convey meaning if the receiver understands them. This is both obvious and frequently overlooked by senders of messages. Students often complain of teachers using abstract concepts and jargon to express meaning which 'goes over the head'. Nurses are sometimes asked after a doctor's visit to explain to patients what was said to them, i.e. to translate technical language into an intelligible form for those without such language. Part of becoming a nurse is being initiated into the concepts and ideas of a body of medical knowledge and to be able to use such language to communicate effectively to other professionals. It is also important to be able to keep the common touch.

Some people consciously (and unconsciously) use language to mystify, impress, dominate, humiliate and to give markers of their social position (see Chapter 3). This use of language is an example of sending multiple messages in which the surface meaning is secondary in importance to the disguised meaning. It is a common enough experience to be in the company of people whose use of technical language defines the boundaries of the group and excludes others. It is noticeable on some professional social occasions that there are forces around to unite groups who use a common language and to exclude others who may find the experience tiresome as a result. 'In-groups', like teenagers, need to keep language on the move with 'in-words' to mark the boundary between 'in' and 'out'.

Given that hearing is the sense that receives the lexical content in speech, a hearing loss is a severe impairment in face-to-face communication. Sign language of the deaf substitutes the sight channel for the hearing channel but is less symbolically rich. Counsellors of the deaf report how much more difficult it is to engage with the nuance and subtleties of feeling in their clients with hearing disabilities compared with clients who can hear. Also, sound carries in three dimensional space—we can hear messages from any direction—whereas the eyes receive from the front only. However, the lexical content is only part of the transmitted message received by hearing; there is also non-verbal communication.

Para-linguistic features

These are the features of a spoken message that are not contained in the words alone i.e. rhythm, pace, emphasis, intonation, pitch and tone of voice. A message such as 'I'll see you at 8 o'clock' can be a simple declaration or a question, depending on the intonation. Emphasis, pace and tone of voice can also make this into an authoritative bark or a seductive invitation.

Such features help in the interpretation of a message by giving the receiver clues about the sender's state of mind. Is she being angry, suspicious, sarcastic, serious, or funny? Loudness, stress and quality of voice encode some of these aspects of communication. The sentence 'She's really caring' can have quite different meanings depending on which word is stressed and contextual clues are likely to reinforce the intended meaning. Accent and dialect can show social class and regional origins and differences. It is impressive to note how much information passes between two people by these para-linguistic features from a single short utterance. In telephone conversations they are particularly important because visual clues from the other person are missing.

Activity 1.1 An exercise in para-linguistic features
Take a simple sentence such as 'I'll see you in the library this afternoon' and, with a partner, experiment to see how many variations in meaning you can achieve simply by changing the way you say the words without actually altering any of them.
What can you deduce from this exercise?

Body language

These two words suggest that there is another channel for carrying meaning and communicating which does not use words at all. Body language has become a popular topic both in everyday conversation and in serious scientific studies of animal and human interaction. As every parent knows, a baby communicates effectively, if imprecisely, both its urgent needs and satisfactions through the use of gestures and non-verbal cries and noises. Each individual, through her own development, can be seen to recapitulate the human race's evolutionary past and this is true also of the development of communication—from gestures and actions, to meaningful grunts and noises, to more articulated sounds which eventually become the language. Visual signals also carry significant meaning and can replace, supplement or contradict a verbal message. Certain hand gestures, for example, are potent messages of affection or contempt and exist across many cultures in different forms. Car drivers, in particular, are subjected to enough of these gestures to be kept up to date on what is currently in vogue.

Dimbleby & Burton (1992) suggest that body language has several elements.

Gesture

While people are speaking they gesture with their hands, some more than others. They provide useful information as experiments have shown in which people describe shapes or movements with or without using their hands (Argyle 1992). More subtle gestures include the steepling of the fingers to express confidence, and listeners often use head nods of different amplitude—small ones to show attention, larger and repeated ones to show agreement. Interestingly, gestures and speech are controlled by the same area of the brain and develop in children at about the same time.

Facial expressions

Possibly because of their important survival value in infancy, subtle variations in smile or look are readily distinguished, especially those located around the eyes and mouth. Whether a listener is pleased, puzzled or annoyed can be detected by observing the eyes and mouth.

Gaze

It follows that gaze is important in assessing non-verbal clues. Gaze is closely coordinated with speech: the speaker usually looks at the listener before making a major grammatical break and particularly before the end of utterances. Speakers often look away when they start to speak or are thinking about what they are saying.

Posture

The way the body is held gives a general indication of confidence, attention, boredom, confrontation and other specific reactions. In western culture people normally stand with their bodies slightly averted from each other when having a conversation to indicate polite friendliness or neutrality. Other cultures have different codes of behaviour and this can be disconcerting sometimes, leading to misunderstandings and even offence.

Body space and proximity

People need a certain space around them to feel comfortable and this varies depending on age, sex and culture. Being squashed into a small space with other people in a lift or a crowded bus generally engenders feelings of awkwardness and discomfort with some relief when personal space is restored. Adults keep an arm's reach away from other people unless they know them reasonably well. It follows that the tensions involved for both parties when a nurse is physically handling and treating a patient are to be expected and need to be acknowledged.

Touch

This tells a good deal about the nature of a relationship and the degree of friendliness between two people. It can also be used as a marker of status, the higher status person implying 'I can touch you but you should not touch me'. Touch is a potent carrier of messages as lovers, friends, relatives and victims of sexual harassment or abuse know. Clearly, different rules of behaviour exist in the medical world from those in everyday life. The traditional view has, perhaps unconsciously, taken heed of this potency by insisting on keeping an emotional distance between carer and patient. A gynaecological examination rarely has eye contact between doctor and patient during the process as if to suggest that to have eye contact as well as body contact would be emotionally too much. Conversely, those treatments which encourage a strong emotional attachment between carer and patient, e.g. psychotherapy, are those in which physical contact is normally regarded as unethical.

Dress

The manner and presentation of dress, hair, jewellery and make-up say a lot about an individual's personality, role, job, status and mood. The use of a uniform is itself a strong statement that the role is more important than the individual. Nurses in some work settings may decide against wearing a uniform following discussions about the intended nature of the relationship between nurse and patient. Individuals in hospital hierarchies often code their position by different forms of dress.

Argyle found that when a stranger behaved in a friendly non-verbal style it created a much more friendly impression than the use of friendly words. He suggests several non-verbal signals that are effective in communicating a friendly attitude (see Box 1.3).

The visual, audible, verbal and non-verbal messages are normally presented together in face-to-face communication. Consistency is sought between the multiple channels with integration of all the information for the fullest picture. If, however, someone says 'I'm *not* angry' but bangs down her fist, the gesture perceived is often taken as the reliable source of information. Conflict and defensiveness are often expressed in such discrepant ways. In general, the verbal message is easier to manipulate and control than the non-verbal message because the first requires conscious processing whilst the latter is usually unconscious. A nurse may intuitively know that

a patient is distressed even though the patient has just said 'I'm all right' because non-verbal messages have been sent and received in clear contradiction of the words uttered. In counselling and psychotherapy a client will frequently tell a grim story with either no emotional tone or with a smile. This discrepancy indicates that the feeling content of the message is difficult to express or 'face'.

THE SENDER AND RECEIVER

The model of communication given earlier makes a clear distinction between processes happening within a person (essentially unobservable) and behaviour that is emitted by a person (public and observable). The emitted behaviour is the content and channel of the message being sent between sender and receiver. Consideration is now given to how a person's behaviour (external world—interpersonal) is linked to her experience of thoughts and feelings (internal world—intrapsychic). The relationship between behaviour and experience is subtle and far-reaching and some of the ideas about the inner world of the person must be explored.

THE PERSONAL INTERNAL WORLD

Psychodynamic theory addresses the intrapsychic world of the person and formulates concepts and ideas to describe and explain it. The first idea is that the forces which shape any human life belong not only to the present—the here and now—but also in the past, especially the distant past i.e. the early life of childhood and even babyhood. A second idea is that human behaviour is best explained in terms of mental processes that are not only unobservable to outsiders but that are also to a large extent unknowable to the individual i.e. they are unconscious. This latter idea provides rich insights into the subtleties and difficulties of human communication. It enables common experiences in communication to be addressed, for example:

Box 1.3	The non-verbal signals of a friendly attitude (from Argyle 1992)
proximity:	closer, lean forward if seated
orientation:	more direct, but side to side for some situations
gaze:	more gaze and mutual gaze
facial expression:	more smiling
gestures:	head nods, lively movements
posture:	open arms stretched towards each other rather than arms on hips or folded
touch:	more touch in an appropriate manner
tone of voice:	higher pitch, upward contour, pure tone
verbal contents:	more self-disclosure

- Understanding the words that someone has said but also having a vague yet strong intuition that there is another unsaid message, often of an emotional sort. Feelings of confusion, bewilderment and unease are not uncommon in such circumstances.
- The way in which individuals have their own code of expression, especially when strong negative emotions are aroused. A person treated appallingly by a colleague might say 'It wasn't a very nice thing to do'. Such idio-syncrasies of expression need to be understood and acknowledged if the full force of a communication is to be appreciated.
- Receiving attacks on one's capacity to comm-unicate and have peace of mind especially from patients who are, either temporarily or chronically, emotionally disturbed. Segal (1991) says that her own observations have shown how clearly a sense of one's own goodness and worth seems to depend on physical health so it is not surprising that people are often emotionally disturbed when they become patients—a fact which is often denied by health professionals.

Some light can be thrown on such common everyday experiences by focusing on the remarkable ability of the human mind to express itself simultaneously on two distinct and yet related levels of meaning. People often express themselves in a single, direct way without any hint of a second meaning. At other times there is a shift to a more complex way of functioning in which encoded messages are generated that have both a surface meaning and a disguised meaning (see Fig. 1.4).

The shift from one form of expression to the other can be quite conscious. One thing is often said which deliberately means something else. If, however, circumstances are highly emotionally charged, either internally or in the outside world, then the shift from one form of expression to the other is beyond conscious control and multiple level messages are deployed unconsciously.

Taken together, a more complex picture of communication emerges in which a person's inner world—the intra-psychic domain—is interacting with any interpersonal messages that are being exchanged. It is because of this interaction that each person has enormous resources for subtle and complex communication with others. It is these resources that can keep friendships and other intimate relationships alive for a lifetime.

To summarise, it is part of normal human development to:

- give surface messages with direct and simple meaning;
- consciously encode a secondary message below the surface message where indirectness is intended; and
- unconsciously deal with difficult emotional situations by encoding messages in disguised form without being aware of doing so.

These three modes of communication from everyday life can now be examined in more detail together with a fourth, commonly known as 'dumping'.

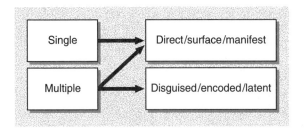

Figure 1.4   Single and multiple levels of communication

Box 1.4   Four modes of communication

1. Surface messages with direct and simple meaning.
2. Consciously encoded messages which contain a secondary message below the surface.
3. Unconsciously encoded messages in which feelings are unconsciously disguised to protect the individual from a disturbing experience/ emotion.
4. 'Dumping' whereby an individual gets rid of disturbing experiences/emotions by dumping them on to someone else.

Direct surface messages

Direct surface messages are vital for survival and depend on logic and reason for their content and form. Many human transactions in the medical world depend on reliable information being transmitted from one person to another without ambiguity or distortion. The safe treatment of a patient is built upon such communication. 'Give this patient 10 milligrams twice a day' and 'Pass me the spatula' are examples of the common occurrence of medical communication that makes any treatment possible. Meaning is clear and the use of language, given a common understanding by sender and receiver of vocabulary and grammar, is limited to dealing with direct surface messages. It is disturbing to the receiver in these circumstances not to understand what is being said, either at the lexical level (not knowing the meaning of a word) or by an unfamiliar use of intonation, accent or dialect. Difficulties are located in the message itself, not in the decoding of the sender's intention. Context has the power to change the surface meaning of even the simplest message. 'I'll kill you if you do that' will be interpreted differently when said with a threatening knife or during a playful episode.

Surface messages have utility, hence their importance, but little else. Conversation in the interpersonal realm is rather bleak if it is made up of surface messages only because all is clear— there is no allusion or implication to stimulate the imagination. In the TV series Star Trek, Mr Spock is infuriating at times to Captain Kirk because of the computer-like logic of his conversation.

Conscious encoding

If the surface message is part of a multiple level message then, to be effective, it must not only be understood on its own terms but also point to a hidden meaning suitably encoded and disguised. The power of great poems, plays or novels stems from their capacity to engage imaginatively at the surface level but also to point to mysterious underlying levels of coded messages that are sensed rather than understood.

In everyday life, deliberate encoding is often employed when tact, consideration and sensi-

tivity are desirable and when a direct message is inadvisable. Painful messages are often expressed through such encoding and the main function of this type of message is to soften the blow, to take advantage of all the means available whereby something is better not fully said. The medical world is full of situations in which painful messages have to be given to patients or their relatives and yet there seems some reluctance to examine, in human terms, the process of giving such a message. (Kubler-Ross 1970.)

Box 1.5 shows an everyday conversation between hospital staff in which both parties consciously encode their messages in the hope of achieving desired results. The sister makes two statements of fact which carry an uncomfortable message for the nurse who struggles to defend herself from the implications using equally encoded messages.

People vary in their responsiveness to encoded messages. The underlying raw message can be avoided by pretending it does not exist. This is often an attempt to frustrate the sender of the encoded communication, attack the intended meanings and preclude any further creative communication along the hidden lines. Another approach is to confront the disguise and to state the 'unsaid' message directly. This is likely to be received as tactless because such a strategy does not respect the need for the encoding in the first place. Perhaps the most common coping method is to register the hidden meaning and to make an appropriate encoded response in return as the nurse does in the example in Box 1.5.

Activity 1.2   An exercise in conscious encoding

Think of situations in which your superior gave you a derivative encoded message together with a surface message. How did you respond? How would you give such a message if the roles were reversed?

Box 1.5   Consciously encoded messages: an example

Sister: What with staff shortages and a holiday coming up I don't know how we are going to cope.
Nurse: I've already worked two double shifts this week.
Sister: I'll be on duty throughout the Bank Holiday.
Nurse: Yes, I know. I covered for Jenny the other day when she was off sick.

Unconscious encoding

This is far too big a subject to be treated in anything but an outline form here. Individuals learn from childhood to protect themselves from dangerous emotions by unconsciously avoiding them and communicating in messages distant from the threatening feelings yet derived from them. A patient may be full of bluster and bravado and be quite unaware that she is afraid.

Activity 1.3   An exercise in unconscious encoding
Think of examples of ways in which patients have unconsciously disguised their feelings in order to protect themselves from disturbing experiences.
How have you been able to relate the inferences from their behaviour to the hidden underlying message?

Such unconscious encoding is universal and it is useful for health professionals to be aware of the general indicators which point to hidden, derivative messages from patients. Considerable caution needs to be applied when trying to understand unconscious messages: it is easy to over-interpret and to misread a straightforward communication. It is also inevitable that the receiver will project personal issues into the communication, at least to some extent, and so contaminate the sender's message. Conversely, there is also the danger that a communication will be taken at face value when, in reality, an important encoded message is being sent which is consequently missed.

There are many clues to suggest someone is sending an encoded message:

- The message may not seem entirely logical, realistic or complete. Clearly many factors have to be considered in order to reach this conclusion—the wider context, the trigger for the communication—and such evaluation should be tentative and should seek validation from other sources.
- There may be contradictions in the communication flow so that one element does not fit in with the general theme(s) and this is noticed by the receiver.

- There may be a discrepancy between how the sender intended the message to be received and understood and how it is actually received. This is the area that most needs external validation if the personal bias of the receiver is not to dominate the interpretation.
- The sender may make inexplicable errors e.g. misperceptions, lapses of memory, behaviour that seems out of keeping with conscious thoughts and intentions, slips of the tongue etc.
- Strong feelings and highly emotional situations are likely to evoke encoded messages with important hidden meanings. This is true where conflict and anxiety are strongly present and also where there is a sense of danger or mistrust.
- The presence of psychosomatic symptoms— phobias, obsessions, anxiety—is another clue to emotional disturbance and the presence of hidden messages.

These indicators of the presence of unconscious encoding of messages need to be assessed with caution. However, given that the health care context is likely to foster the use of messages with important encoded meanings, it can help genuine communication considerably if health professionals are aware of this dimension to ordinary human contact.

Dumping

Any attempt to define communication would be incomplete without addressing a familiar experience in human interaction, commonly known as dumping. When dumping, individuals are not concerned with communicating meaning but with getting rid of feelings or something disturbing within themselves—an evacuation process.

The goal of the dumper is either to discharge internal discomfort by creating a comparable disturbance in the receiver (an unconscious wish 'I'll make you feel as bad as I do'), or to get the receiver to incorporate the disturbance to see how she deals with it ('I'll put my bad feelings into you and see how you cope with it'). Nurses frequently report experiences with patients that make them feel agitated and upset. The patient offloads disturbing feelings on to the nurse who subsequently feels 'dumped' into and exploited as if she is carrying the discomfort that was originally with the patient.

For some individuals the desire to rid themselves of inner disturbance goes alongside a desire to understand their inner and interpersonal struggles. Once dumping is over they can take part in a quieter form of meaningful communication and explore underlying issues. There are others who want only to get rid of what disturbs them and to upset the receiver. They are neither interested in understanding what they are doing and why, nor are they concerned for the effect which the dumping may have on the receiver.

Dumping is a maladaptive means of communicating. It is focussed on action and discharge rather than reflection and creates alienation and antagonism. It is not uncommon for a known dumper, whether patient or colleague, to clear the social space of listeners as soon as she appears! Dumping can bring no lasting comfort to the dumper because this method of communicating cannot enhance growth, learning or reflection. Dumpers are prisoners of their communication style and endlessly repeat the dumping process in a vain attempt to secure relief from internal tension.

Finally, it is important to recognise our own dumping tendencies and to manage and contain them from our own internal resources. In addition, the ability to recognise dumping tendencies in others can foster effective communicative reactions within ourselves, which otherwise would lead to communicative misunderstanding and alienation.

FINAL MODEL OF COMMUNICATION

We are now in a position to represent some of this complexity in a final diagram (see Fig. 1.5).

This takes account of the fact that there are probably an enormous number of messages flowing between those involved in one-to-one

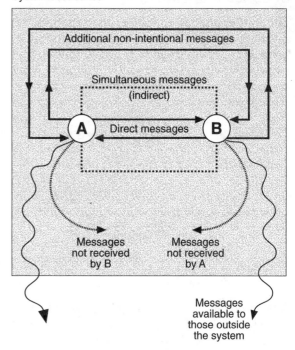

System boundaries

Figure 1.5 A model of communication (taken from Ellis & McClintock 1990)

communication: some messages never get through to the receiver; some are disregarded even when they do get through; and some messages are perceived only by those outside the interaction.

CONCLUSION

This chapter has taken a broad look at the nature of face-to-face human communication: direct, indirect, conscious, unconscious and dumping. Like so many other aspects of human life, communication becomes more complicated the closer it is examined and our definition of the word should now be much broader than might have been expected at the outset. In the next chapter we look closely at the person in communication, i.e. the sender and receiver of messages, and use the theoretical ideas of psychologists to further develop our view of human communication.

REFERENCES

Argyle M 1992 The social psychology of everyday life. Routledge, London.

Bateson G, Jackson D D, Haley J, Weakland J 1956 Toward a theory of schizophrenia. Behavioural Science 1:251.

Bradley J C, Edinberg M A 1990 Communication in the nursing context, 3rd edn. Appleton and Lange, Connecticut.

Dimbleby R, Burton G 1992 More than words: an introduction to communication, 2nd edn. Routledge, London.

Ellis R, McClintock A 1990 If you take my meaning. Arnold, London.

Kubler-Ross E 1970 On death and dying. Tavistock/ Routledge, London.

Laing R D 1959 The divided self. Tavistock, London.

Langs R 1983 Unconscious communication in everyday life. Jason Aronson, New York.

Menzies-Lyth I 1960 The functioning of social systems as a defence against anxiety. In: Containing anxiety in institutions 1988. Free Association Books, London.

Segal J 1991 The use of the concept of unconscious phantasy in understanding reactions to chronic illness. In: Counselling, November 1991.

Watzlawick P, Beavin J, Jackson D 1967 Pragmatics of human communication. Norton, New York.

FURTHER READING

Berryman J 1987 Psychology and you. Methuen, London.

Burton G, Dimbleby R 1988 Between ourselves. Arnold, London.

Cooper C L 1986 Improving interpersonal relations. Wildwood House, Aldershot.

Hein E C 1980 Communication in nursing practice, 2nd edn. Little, Brown, Boston.

Morrison P, Burnard P 1991 Caring and communicating. Macmillan, London.

Wainwright G R 1985 Body language. Hodder and Stoughton, Kent.

2

The person in communication

Roger Ellis
Robert J. Gates

INTRODUCTION

The previous chapter looked at the nature of communication and compiled a complex picture based on the simple definition of sender, message, receiver. We emphasised the message, its nature, its capacity to have single and multiple meanings and the ways in which it could be sent and received. In this chapter we focus on the sender and receiver, i.e. on the persons who are communicating. To understand the meaning of a message, assumptions are necessarily made about the person who sent it. This is true not only of an individual person but also of people in general.

The link between communication and assumptions about people can be frequently observed. Children are often treated as if they do not understand what is happening around them when they quite clearly do. People with a physical disability often complain about bizarre assumptions made of them, for example, that they are deaf or unintelligent. The bedside communication between a doctor and a nurse in a hospital situation might reveal to the patient their assumptions about the role of a sick person. The power of role and context to determine the nature of communication is examined in more detail in Chapter 3.

In order to examine what these general underlying assumptions might be and in order to assess alternatives, we need first to have some knowledge of the theory of human nature. People observe other people and develop theories about why others behave as they do and how they are different. For professional carers it is necessary to have some means of predicting how people are going to behave in general even if each is treated as an individual. Effective caring practice is built on coherent theory which is itself built on basic assumptions. Actions need to be grounded in theory if they are not to be random and incoherent. For practice to be more effective, we need to make explicit the underlying assumptions and theory which otherwise remain implicit and hidden.

PSYCHODYNAMIC, BEHAVIOURIST AND HUMANISTIC THEORY

There are three theoretical approaches to the person in communication which are commonly used in a nursing context—the psychodynamic, the behaviourist and the humanistic theories. Each has arisen in a particular context for a particular purpose and each makes a significant contribution to an understanding of the complexity of human nature. In this chapter we concentrate on the different basic concepts, principles, assumptions and applicability of each theory. Individuals will then be in a position to compare their own personal theory-making with that of other specialists in the field, and potentially gain new insights into communication with others.

WHAT DIVIDES THE THEORISTS?

There are six basic issues which divide theorists (Pervin, 1993) and which reflect the personal life experiences of the theorists as well as the social and scientific trends current at the time of their work (see Box 2.1). The way in which these issues are addressed affects the way in which a person is viewed and which aspects of human functioning are chosen for emphasis and investigation.

The philosophical view

People rarely need to articulate to each other the values and beliefs that underlie their view of the world. Any coherent theory of the person is built upon a philosophical view concerning human

---

Box 2.1   Six basic issues to divide theorists (Pervin, 1993)

1. The philosophical view of the person.
2. The relation between internal (personal) and external (situational) influences in determining behaviour.
3. The concept of the self and how to account for organised functioning.
4. The role of varying states of awareness.
5. The relationships between feeling, thought and behaviour.
6. The role of the past, present and future in governing behaviour.

---

nature. One theory emphasises instinctive forces, another social factors. Are people driven or are they free? Rational or compulsively irrational? Self-seeking or capable of altruism? Spiritual or biological beings? These issues and many others have been debated throughout history and are at the root of any major shift in the perception and treatment of patients receiving medical care.

When seeking to understand a philosophical model it is useful to consider its philosophical base. The model that best suits an individual will be influenced by personal factors, life experiences, culture and by the spirit of the times, just as the original proponents of each model were so influenced. The psychodynamic model—with its origins in Freud's ideas—views the person as a product of early experiences. Skinner's (1938) behaviourist view believes behaviour is a response to the environment and the feedback received from it. Carl Rogers' (1970) humanistic, or person-centred view is that each individual is a self-actualising organism which has a basically positive drive towards health and happiness.

Internal and external forces

A second and related issue is whether the causes of behaviour are inside a person or outside in the environment. The extreme views are easy to recognise. Freud believes human beings are controlled by unknown internal forces within the unconscious, whereas Skinner suggests that a person does not act upon the world, the world acts upon him, i.e. he is controlled by environmental forces. To a certain extent all views are interactive but it is worth asking whether the focus of any one view is on internal, personal factors or on external, environmental factors.

The concept of self

To be a distinct person is to have some coherent, consistent pattern and organisation of thought, feeling and behaviour. To account for this aspect of human functioning the concept of self has been used. Awareness of self is an important part of experience. The way individuals feel about themselves affects their outlook on the world and their behaviour towards others. Theorists differ considerably in their use of the self. Rogers makes it the central integrating concept as the person seeks to make the self and experience congruent with each other. Skinner in principle avoids the very notion of self as a vague, romantic and fanciful idea.

Awareness and consciousness

It is generally recognised by psychologists that the potential exists for different states of consciousness in human experience. Nevertheless, there is strong disagreement as to whether the concept of the unconscious is useful or necessary to explain the diverse phenomena of experience. How are dreams accounted for? Can people give an accurate account of themselves or are large parts of their thoughts, feelings and behaviour outside their awareness? The answers to these and other questions determine how people communicate and how they interpret what is said. If a nurse asks a patient how he is feeling does she take the answer to be the truth of the matter or are other factors to be taken into account?

Thoughts, feelings and behaviour

Theorists differ in the relative weight they give to each of these areas of functioning. From the psychodynamic view all behaviour is a product of thought and feeling. Behaviourists focus on overt behaviour and reject any investigation of internal processes. Other theorists argue that thoughts are primary and cause both feelings and behaviour. Still others argue that emotions are primary and can direct thought and behaviour. Although there is a growing acceptance that all three aspects influence each other, the relative emphasis of one over the others distinguishes one model of the person from another.

The past, present and future

Is behaviour determined by the past or by expectations of the future, or solely by factors in the present? This is yet another issue that divides theorists. The distinguishing feature in each of the different theories is how the links between all three—past, present and future—are conceptualised. If people are viewed as being determined by their past with little hope for change they are unlikely to be treated differently, with a more optimistic view of the future. A nurse's whole basis for communication with a patient is built on his view of the relation between the present state of affairs and a prospective future.

Having examined the basic issues that divide theorists, the three models can be examined in more detail.

THE PSYCHODYNAMIC MODEL

The psychodynamic understanding of the person is derived from the work of Sigmund Freud. His theories and techniques of psychoanalysis have provided a rich source of ideas that many others have since developed and modified. This has given rise to a vast and complex literature involving many different schools of thought which can be confusing and overwhelming to a new reader.

The word 'psychodynamic' is a useful one because it refers not to one theory only but to the many theories that owe their origins to the pioneering work of Freud. The two parts to the word offer some insight into the focus of the model. 'Psyche' is sometimes understood as mind but is best seen as referring to the whole of a person's inner world of feelings, thoughts and

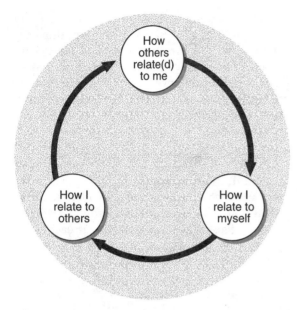

Figure 2.1 The external becomes internal becomes external

experiences. Older words such as soul and spirit need to be added to do justice to the word 'psyche'. 'Dynamic' refers to the view that the psyche is seen as active and not static, not only relating to other people but also active within itself, relating to itself. Reflection on experience and the way we describe experience, e.g. 'I just did it. I don't know why. I feel so cross with myself' often reveals a person's internal relationships which are full of feeling and are not necessarily linked to other people at all. Thus the dynamic is both internal and external and the word 'psychodynamic' applies to the internal world of experience which in turn affects the external world. The way in which we relate to ourselves—with compassion, hatred, fear or envy—is expressed outside in the way we relate to others. Hence our style of communicating with others is derived from our communication with ourselves (see Fig. 2.1).

OBJECT RELATIONS THEORY

Freud's original theory emphasised the instinctive drives of the individual alone. Object Relations theory, a development from Freud, puts centre-stage the need of human beings to relate to each other and shows how early relationships become internalised and repeated in the ways in which a person relates to himself and others. The term 'object' is somewhat confusing initially because it refers usually to persons and relationships rather than things. The basic assumptions of the psychodynamic Object Relations model of the person are concisely given by Noonan (1983) in Box 2.2 and are briefly described below.

Product and author

Individuals are generally viewed as products of the environment and the time and place in history. People develop conceptions about themselves, about whether they are lovable, clever and good-looking, or unlovable, stupid and ugly. These perceptions enable the person to make sense of the world and make it predictable. An expectation of being rejected will affect the interaction with the next unfamiliar person we meet. This tendency will result in the achievement of the 'self-fulfilling prophecy'.

Harder to accept is the fact that these adult feelings and behaviours have roots in the much earlier experiences of childhood and infancy. Patterns of relating to our earliest figures, usually

---

Box 2.2 Basic assumptions of the psychodynamic model (after Noonan 1983)

1. Each individual is the product and author of his own particular history: how he is now is a direct consequence of his earliest experiences with others and his environment. Subsequent experience confirms or modifies that early experience, for better or worse. He is not, however, passive in his history, but contributes to its shape.
2. He lives simultaneously in his external and internal worlds: the former he is mostly aware of, but the latter is primarily unconscious. The unconscious, internal world is energetic and substantially determines his feelings and actions in the external world.
3. All behaviour, no matter how apparently irrational and senseless, is logical and purposeful according to some personal system.
4. Chronological growth is inexorable, but emotional growth is beset by anxieties and detoured by defences and so doesn't always keep pace. Emotional disturbance is likely to be caused by some outdated and no longer appropriate motivation, decision (defence) or wish.

parents, are internalised resulting in an internal world that is dominated by feelings of anxiety and fear, or of confidence and worth. These early experiences are beyond normal memory, leaving unconscious constructions and expectations about later life. Conscious and deliberate interpretations are made about what is happening in the present and these factors actively contribute to shaping behaviour. Individuals are both product and author of their own history.

Those in the medical profession often have to live with the tension of ambivalent feelings towards a patient. Knowing that to some extent patients are victims of circumstances arouses a desire to help and serve the patient's best interests by understanding and compassion. However, it is common to see quite clearly how much a patient is contributing to his present condition, sometimes consciously but often quite unconsciously. It is difficult for a patient to hold both 'product and author' in mind and to take some appropriate responsibility for his present condition. It is also difficult for carers when the patient will not take responsibility and will not cooperate. The examples in Box 2.3 give illustrations of this tension.

External and internal worlds

The second assumption makes the reality of the unconscious mind a centrepiece. It can safely be said that the unravelling of the workings of the unconscious was one of Freud's major contributions to understanding the human person. All sorts of things can be unconscious: drives, wishes, conflicts, fears, values, aims, defences, images of people and the self, and relationships.

Box 2.3 Patients being products and authors

One of the recent debates in medicine has been centred on whether a doctor is justified in refusing to operate on patients with heart conditions who refuse to stop smoking. The moral dilemma rests on whether the doctor is obliged to treat the patient without his cooperation even though the treatment may be less effective as a result or whether the doctor should choose patients who do accept responsibility for their condition and are prepared to act accordingly.

The issue of suicide and euthanasia involves allied considerations of responsibility.

Psychodynamic theorists such as Klein (1963) suggest that unconscious phantasy underlies all thinking and feeling, not just the feelings of conscious awareness. Such phantasy begins very early in childhood and is primarily concerned with bodily processes and relating to others. It becomes more and more symbolic and elaborate during growth and development but it never loses its primitive roots in infancy. Phantasies about being abandoned, lost or heroically saved, for example, seem to exist independently of whether any of these things actually happened in reality. They appear to be products of the mind rather than of direct experience even though such events do also actually happen.

This internal world constantly interacts with the external one and people live simultaneously in both . When both worlds are in harmony there are no problems in living. It is when the conscious and unconscious wishes and aims differ that conflict and confusion are experienced. If the boundary between the two worlds becomes blurred it is possible to misconstrue people and events in potentially disastrous ways. The unconscious internal world is energetic because of its origins in infancy and when it surfaces it does so with the force of infantile feeling that can be highly disturbing. Box 2.4 gives examples of these points.

All behaviour is logical

The third assumption asserts that all behaviour has meaning if looked for. What appears to be bizarre behaviour in the present is usually derived from the demands of the unconscious breaking through the defence structure, from patterns of long ago in childhood, or as a result of living in a permanently defensive way. At some time in the past coping strategies may have been necessary and comforting but are now anachronistic. The present behaviour derived from them now seems senseless or maladaptive but if the whole historic picture were to be known it would make sense. The term defence is used to refer to the ways in which the human psyche has evolved to protect itself from the feelings of anxiety that inevitably arise from unconscious forces. Box 2.5 gives a list of common defence mechanisms.

Box 2.4 Intrusion of the unconscious into conscious life

Patients often relate to nurses in a way that is not typical of adult functioning but reveals early emotional attachments. The 'good' nurse is one who cares and to care is to do all that the patient requests. A 'bad' nurse is one who is not absolutely devoted to the well-being of the patient and who has to deal with others too. Attitudes to different nurses often have this split quality in which one can do no wrong and another can do no right. Klein suggests that this is the way in which babies relate to their mothers—mother is either all good or all bad—and in the case below this is the way the patient is relating unconsciously to the nurses.

Helen has one patient on her ward, Mrs A, who relates to her in highly unpredictable ways. She never knows what is awaiting her when she comes on duty. On one occasion Mrs. A goes on at length about how wonderful Helen is and what an ideal nurse she makes. At another, Helen is attacked and upbraided for her unfeeling neglect of Mrs. A who seems mortally wounded if Helen has to attend to someone else. Helen finds these violent swings of mood difficult to deal with and tends to reduce contact with Mrs A to a minimum.

Klein suggests that such ruthless use of the nurse as either an ideal object or a completely bad object is typical of early patterns of relating and can be assumed to be unconscious in Mrs A.

Box 2.5 Common defence mechanisms

1. Repression: Unconscious exclusion of memories, feelings etc. from awareness in order to prevent anxiety or guilt.
2. Denial: protecting oneself from painful reality by a refusal to recognise anxiety-provoking elements.
3. Displacement: transferring feelings or actions from their original target to another object that arouses less anxiety.
4. Reaction formation: disguising unconscious motivation by behaving in the opposite way.
5. Projection: attributing one's own (undesirable) traits to other people or agencies.
6. Intellectualisation: masking anxiety-arousing feelings by discussing them in a detached, intellectual manner.
7. Rationalisation: devising apparently rational, socially approved reasons for one's behaviour.

Such defence mechanisms have a positive aspect in that they help the individual control and understand emotional experiences. When defences are down the person may be unable to function and feel overwhelmingly vulnerable. Defence mechanisms, however, also have a negative aspect when they are so strong that they make it difficult to act spontaneously or with trust. Thus potentially rewarding experiences may be inaccessible to the overdefensive person.

Emotional development

The fourth assumption points to the fact that the growth linked to the passage of time, such as physical development and ageing, has a given and irreversible quality about it. Emotional development on the other hand is not linear or steady and has many a detour and reversal. The term 'fixation' is applied if emotional development stops altogether and 'regression' if there is a reversion to an earlier state or way of functioning. Patients frequently show regressive behaviour i.e. they act and feel as though they were much younger, especially when they are stressed, as they often are when ill. Being helpless and dependent may make the strongest of patients feel so anxious that he may well regress to a more infantile state and is then likely to feel the other anxieties of that stage, such as unrealistic fears of danger or abandonment.

The psychodynamic model of the person uses many concepts that have found their way into everyday language but which are here used in a more technical and restricted way, e.g. phantasy, defence and regression. Another important concept is transference. This is the process by which one person unconsciously relates to another in present circumstances in ways that are derived from the past. A nurse, for example, might react to a doctor as if he were his mother. He may know that the doctor is not at all like his mother but nevertheless find himself having familiar feelings whenever the doctor talks to or looks at him. See Box 2.6 for an illustration.

APPLICATION AND LIMITATION

The psychodynamic concepts and assumptions outlined here interrelate to give a coherent picture of the person. Such a view is helpful when communication with or from others has a component of indirectness, of something alluded to but not made explicit, as outlined in Chapter 1.

Box 2.6   Illustration of transference at work

Diane, the eldest of four children, remembers her childhood as one in which her mother was never quite available for her emotionally. She always seemed to be busy with something or somebody else who Diane felt was more important then she was. Diane had an unconscious phantasy that if only she could do more for her mother and be a good little helper and carer she would receive the attention from her mother that she longed for.

From an early age, Diane had chosen nursing as her career. She threw herself into her training and her job and all was well for a while. Then she began to feel that other people's needs were like demands that she could not refuse and therefore resented and for which Diane felt she never received adequate recognition. A vicious circle developed in which Diane became more and more attentive and more and more tired and resentful. It was after a considerable period of guilt and depressive feelings that Diane realised painfully that her motives for coming into nursing had more to do with her unresolved relationship with her mother than with actually caring for the well-being of patients. She had transferred into the work situation, initially quite unconsciously, patterns of behaving and relating from her early childhood.

This is an example of what Bowlby (1979) has called 'compulsive care-giving' and what Malan (1979) has called the 'helping profession syndrome'. The person compulsively gives to others what he would like to have for himself which, as Malan notes, leads to 'a severe deficit in the emotional balance of payments'.

When things are straightforward there is no need to resort to the concepts of the unconscious to help explain behaviour. It is worth remembering that ill or stressed patients are likely to behave in ways quite untypical of their normal behaviour and it is useful to have some ideas available that can potentially make sense of what is happening.

Although it can help to be aware of psychic mechanisms in communication with others, a deeper exploration with a patient into his feelings and the meaning of his behaviour is likely to need a great deal of time and skill. This type of help is more the remit of counselling and psychotherapy. Nevertheless, given that treatment of illness and communication with patients is now seen to involve a relationship between patient and carer, it is not surprising that some writers in the field (e.g. Balint 1964) suggest that an understanding of psychodynamic processes is required to effectively treat a person's entire illness rather than the disease or symptoms alone.

It is perhaps now possible for the reader to reexamine the six issues that divide theorists (see Box 2.1) and to identify where the psychodynamic model stands relative to each.

BEHAVIOURISM

At the turn of the century a group of psychologists became dissatisfied with the psychodynamic approach to the explanation and understanding of the person and developed a new school of psychology known as behaviourism. Pivotal to this perspective was the theory that all behaviour rested on learnt responses to given stimuli, often referred to as associative, connectionist or behavioural theory. This relationship between a stimulus and a response by an organism is accounted for by an understanding of both classical and operant conditioning.

THE BEHAVIOURAL MODEL

The behavioural perspective of understanding the person is grounded in early psychological research into the nature of learning. This approach to understanding learning was first postulated by a neurophysiologist called Pavlov who in 1902 described a relationship between unconditioned responses and unconditioned stimuli. The response was called unconditioned because it was almost reflex in nature, meaning that it was an integral component of the organism's repertoire of behaviour. The most famous example of this is the response of salivation by a dog to the presence of food. In a series of experiments on dogs Pavlov found that if an unconditioned stimulus was paired with a conditioned stimulus then it would be possible to elicit a conditioned response. This is demonstrated in Figure 2.2 as occurring in three stages. In Stage 1, the unconditioned stimulus of food causes the dog to respond by salivating. If this unconditioned response (Stage 2) is paired for a sufficient time with a conditioned stimulus (the bell) then eventually the response of salivation can be obtained by using the conditioned

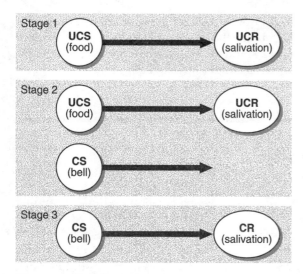

Figure 2.2 Classical conditioning

stimulus alone. That is, the response becomes conditioned to the sound of the bell.

The work of Pavlov was extremely important at the turn of the century in shaping the thinking of the emerging group of American psychologists now referred to as behaviourists. Of these the psychologist, John Watson, became credited as the founder of behaviourism. He believed that in order for psychology to become a science, its data had to be objective and measurable. He was not concerned with introspective, hypothetical causes of behaviour but with public, observable and measurable causes. Watson argued that behaviour was the direct result of conditioning. He believed this conditioning emanated from the environment in which the organism was located and that this environment would shape an organism's behaviour by reinforcing specific behaviours.

He further believed that simple chains of stimulus/response connections formed into longer, more complex strings of behaviour. These

strings of behaviour, he argued, explained how a person thought and what motivated him. In addition, they accounted for personality, emotion, learning and remembering. Such beliefs were clearly articulated by Watson (1924) when he said:

Give me a dozen healthy infants, well-formed, and my own specified world to bring them up in and I'll guarantee to take any one at random and train him to become any kind of specialist I might select—lawyer, artist, merchant, chief and yes even a beggar man and thief, regardless of his talents, penchants, abilities, vocations, and race of his ancestors.

(Watson, 1924)

Such a belief can be seen to be in complete contrast to the psychodynamic approach.

From this early work on behaviourism emerged, amongst others, the work of Skinner (1938). His work, known as operant conditioning, latterly became known as behaviour modification. Skinner's contribution in this area is important because he was the first psychologist to point to the clinical and social relevance of operant conditioning (Bellack et al, 1982). The next section provides examples of the application of behaviourism which has been used as a therapeutic strategy to deal with psychological disorder and to improve or develop communication.

Operant conditioning

Operant conditioning suggests that when an organism makes a connection between a stimulus, the elicited response and the subsequent rewards or punishment, then its behaviour is reinforced either negatively or positively (see Fig. 2.3).

Behaviourists believe that if a behaviour is reinforced positively then the incidence of that behaviour will increase. Conversely, if a behaviour is negatively reinforced the incidence of that behaviour will decrease. The essential

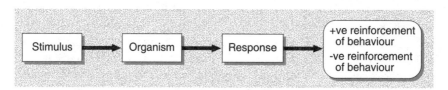

Figure 2.3 Operant conditioning

difference between operant and classical conditioning is that in the latter the behaviour is a part of the animal's repertoire of behaviour. For example, salivation is a naturally occurring response of some organisms to food which can become conditioned by the repeated pairing of a conditioned stimulus (for example a bell) with an unconditioned stimulus (for example food), as described above. In operant conditioning, however, the behaviour is not a part of the animal's repertoire of behaviour. The deliberate or otherwise use of reinforcement will result in a new behaviour.

In 1957, Skinner postulated a behavioural explanation for the acquisition of language in children. He argued that if an infant's vocalising was positively reinforced, then that infant would increase the frequency of that behaviour. Skinner (1957) outlined three ways in which the process of language acquisition might be achieved, as shown in Box 2.7.

Although greatly simplified the process outlined demonstrates how the behavioural model would explain the acquisition of language in order to communicate.

The application of behaviourism

Operant conditioning, as an approach to understanding learning and behaviour, has had an enormous impact upon nursing and the ways in which some client groups are cared for. One behavioural treatment used in the field of mental health, for phobic conditions, is systematic desensitisation. This technique consists of pairing a response that inhibits anxiety, for example muscle relaxation, with something that provokes anxiety. Consider the case of an individual

---

Box 2.7 A behavioural explanation for language acquisition

1. Echoic response: here the infant mimics a noise made by others, who in turn reinforce the infant's behaviour.
2. Mand response: the infant engages in initiating sound but without meaning. The meaning is attached by others, once again reinforcement of the behaviour is provided by others.
3. Tact response: at this stage the child moves on to make an attempt to use a word to name something that is present in its environment. When the child successfully does this its behaviour is reinforced.

---

suffering from arachnophobia (a fear of spiders). In desensitisation a therapist would pair the anxiety-provoking event in a graduated manner with relaxation techniques. So for example the therapist would commence desensitisation by showing the patient a photograph of a spider coupled with relaxation exercises. Eventually the therapist would show the patient a living spider and perhaps get him to touch the spider, again coupled with relaxation exercises. In between these two extremes are a series of graduated stimuli that could cause a corresponding graduated fear response. This is shown in Figure 2.4.

However, repeated pairing of the stimuli with relaxation would eventually bring about a different response to fear at the sight of spiders. Instead a patient would feel more comfortable and relaxed, because they would associate the relaxation with the spider instead of the anxiety and fear.

For a detailed description of this type of therapeutic intervention the reader is advised to see Paul and Bernstein (1976). Bellack (1982) described the use of behaviourism as a mediator

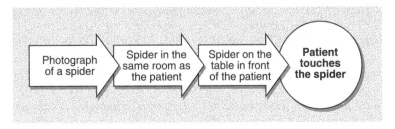

Figure 2.4 Systematic desensitisation

in a number of studies of social skills training for schizophrenic patients. He suggested that social skills were deficient in schizophrenic patients, resulting in social isolation. One study comprised targeting and improving the assertiveness of two chronic schizophrenic patients. Eye contact, speech duration, smiles, requests and compliances were reinforced positively. Results demonstrated that the targeted behaviours significantly improved and that these improvements remained for some weeks after the skills training

Another example of the use of behavioural interventions to improve communication is recorded by Lovass (1976). A series of steps was taken to train autistic children in vocal imitation. In Step 1, the therapist increased the child's vocalisations by reinforcing him (usually with food) contingent on such behaviour. In Step 2, the child was trained in temporal discrimination: his vocalisations were reinforced only if they were in response to the therapist's speech, i.e. if they occurred within five seconds of the therapist's vocalisation. In Step 3, finer discriminations were reinforced. For example, the child was reinforced for making successively closer approximations to the therapist's speech until he could match the particular sound given by the therapist. Lovass (1976) continued with a detailed account of how new behaviour was reinforced leading to increased vocalisation in the children.

The examples given serve to demonstrate how a behaviourist view of the person may influence the ways in which nurses communicate with their patients. McCue (1993) has demonstrated very clearly how the behavioural approach can be used to help people with both learning disabilities and challenging behaviours.

In Table 2.1 the features that characterise the behavioural approach to understanding the person are shown alongside the features of the psychodynamic and humanistic approaches.

Having briefly outlined the behavioural approach to understanding the person let us now consider the third of the three approaches, the humanistic model.

Table 2.1   Characteristics of the psychodynamic, behavioural and humanistic models

Issues	Psychodynamic (O-R) model	Behavioural model	Humanistic model
Philosophical view of the person	Basic drive is to relate to others and things. The person is the author and product of experience.	All behaviour is learned in response to environmental reinforcement.	Positive view of human beings. Drive towards becoming fully functioning.
Internal v. external orientation	Dynamic interaction between inner and outer experience.	Emphasis on external stimuli and measurable behaviour.	Congruence between inner and outer experience is the ideal.
Self concept	Various interpretations and emphases across several workers.	Observable and measurable focus. Therefore self is largely ignored.	Key, central concept. Self is involved in thought, feeling and behaviour.
States of awareness	The unconscious is a central concept. Dynamic interplay between conscious and unconscious processes.	Awareness and insight not central ideas.	Accepts unconscious but focuses on the here and now.
Feeling, thought and behaviour	Dynamic interplay between all three.	Behaviour is central focus.	Felt experience primary. Congruence between all three in the present is the ideal.
Role of past, present and future	Past and present in constant dynamic interaction.	Focus on the present and the future.	Congruence can only be experienced in the present moment.

THE HUMANISTIC MODEL

Atkinson et al (1990) have suggested that during the first half of this century the psychodynamic and behavioural approaches to understanding the person were dominant. However, during the late 1950s and early 1960s a group of psychologists developed a new and radical approach based on phenomenology in which the humanistic approach to understanding the person is central. Phenomenology rejects the behavioural approach to understanding the person where behaviour is seen as the result of associations or connections between stimuli and responses. It also rejects the suggestion that behaviour is controlled by unconscious impulses, located in our past, as suggested by the psychodynamic approach. Instead, humanism asserts the unique, subjective and lived experience of each individual.

From the humanistic approach came the work of Maslow (1954) (see page 75) who describes a system of hierarchy of needs in the person. These needs range from basic physiological needs such as food, water, and air to complex psychological needs such as security, belonging and self-esteem. The pinnacle of this hierarchy is self actualisation: the individual's need to find fulfilment and develop to his own potential. Another important contributor to the humanistic approach is Carl Rogers. His ideas emerged from his therapeutic work with people in need of psychotherapy. He believed that people have an innate tendency to develop and grow in maturity which will lead an individual to actualise all the capacities he has. Central to this approach is a fundamental philosophical belief in the individual to develop to his full potential. Atkinson (1990) offered the four principles outlined in Box 2.8 which characterise the humanistic outlook of the person.

Two excellent examples of how the humanistic approach affects the ways in which nurses and other therapists communicate with people can be found in the specialism of learning disability. It will be seen from the examples given that the principles of humanism affect the type of relationship between the nurse and the person being cared for.

Box 2.8 The four principles of humanism

1. *The person is of central interest.*
   Humanists assert that people are not merely objects that respond to their environment when suitably reinforced. Rather people are dynamic interactive beings who are able to shape their environment as well as respond to it.
2. *Aspects of human behaviour are important to investigation.*
   Central to humanism is the idea of the quest for fulfilment and self actualisation as described by Rogers (1970). Human choice and creativity are important parts of this.
3. *Subjectivity is more important than objectivity.*
   Understanding the lived experience of people is essential. Humanists argue that the rigours of other schools of psychology distort the nature of human experience in the pursuit of objectivity.
4. *The value of the person.*
   Great value is placed upon the integrity and uniqueness of the individual. Humanists believe that the objective of psychology should be to understand the individual and should not be concerned with controlling and manipulating the person.

BEHAVIOURAL DIFFICULTIES AND LEARNING DISABILITIES

The DOH reported in 1992 that within the specialism of learning disability there was a group of people who demonstrated challenging behaviours or mental health needs. The report said:

People with learning disabilities who have challenging behaviours form an extremely diverse group, including individuals with all levels of learning disability, many different sensory or physical impairments and presenting quite different kinds of challenges. The group includes, for example, people with mild or borderline disability who have been diagnosed as mentally ill and who enter the criminal justice system for crimes such as arson or sexual offences; as well as people with profound learning disability, often with sensory handicaps and other physical health problems, who injure themselves, for example by repeated head banging or eye poking.
(DOH 1992)

This operational definition is clearly very broad and in this section we focus specifically on behavioural difficulties. For many years the most dominant forms of therapeutic intervention for behavioural difficulties were based upon behaviourism. That is, therapeutic programmes were developed for individuals that reinforced desirable behaviours and punished or ignored undesirable behaviours. In the early 1980s two researchers (Menolascino & McGee 1991) from the University of Nebraska challenged this approach as inappropriate. They argued that the behavioural approach did not respect the integrity and uniqueness of people with a learning disability who were a devalued group. They promoted instead an enlightened approach that has come to be called Gentle Teaching.

Gentle Teaching

This form of therapeutic intervention comprises a range of strategies that uses non-aversive techniques. The principle aim is to develop bonding between individuals. Unlike behavioural approaches the provision of 'rewards' does not depend upon a demonstration of desirable behaviours sought by the therapist. Gentle Teaching would appear to comprise four core themes outlined in Box 2.9.

It is fair to say that there is considerable debate about the legitimacy and efficacy of such interventions (Jones & Connell 1993). Notwithstanding the criticisms that have been made,

---

Box 2.9   Gentle Teaching: four core themes
1. *Unconditional valuing.* Gentle teaching asserts the importance of valuing the person and the giving of non contingent reinforcement as opposed to behaviourism, where reinforcement is contingent upon desired behaviour. 2. *Teaching the client to value others.* The person is taught to return this unconditional valuing to others, not purely as a response to reinforcement but as part of the interdependence of people. 3. *Changing the attitudes of carers.* Menolascino and McGee recognised the need to change the attitudes of staff caring for people with challenging behaviour to become more enlightened and develop closer bonds between them and the people being cared for. 4. *Human engagement.* Lastly McGee points to the need for meaningful interaction between people that fully engages them, i.e. that human beings need to relate to one another as human beings in committed relationships.

Gentle Teaching is an excellent example of how a particular view or theory of a person impacts upon the ways in which nurses and therapists communicate and interact with people with a learning disability.

Activity 2.1   An exercise in Gentle Teaching
The reader is invited to spend some time reflecting upon Gentle Teaching and then identify those characteristics that suggest its practice and ideology to be grounded in humanism.

Normalisation (social role valorisation)

Wolfensberger (1972) stated that 'people with a mental handicap have the same rights and, wherever possible, the same responsibilities as other people of the same age in any given society' (Wolfensberger 1972). This valuing and enlightened outlook on the individual was clearly in keeping with the humanist perspective of the person. Nowhere were the underlying ideological principles of normalisation more clearly articulated than by Grunewald (1969) who said:

The principle of normalisation is applicable both to the development of the retarded individual [adult or child] and to the needs of parents—the validity of this principle is not negated by the fact that the majority of mentally handicapped persons cannot become fully adjusted to society. The term implies rather a striving in various ways towards what is normal. Even the most severely handicapped person can thus be normalised in one or more respects. Normalisation does not imply any denial of the person's handicap. It involves rather exploiting his other mental and physical capabilities so that his handicap becomes less pronounced. It also means that he has the same rights and obligations as other people, as near as possible.

(Grunewald 1969)

Chisholm (1993) has identified seven core themes of normalisation which are detailed in Box 2.10 and are briefly described below.

The role of consciousness and unconsciousness in service provision. Much of the work of professionals can be conducted on an unconscious level, without sensitivity towards the ways in which their own values affect the nature of interaction and communication with the people they care for. These unconscious values

Box 2.10	The core themes of normalisation

1. The role of consciousness and unconsciousness in services.
2. The relevance of role expectancy and role circularity.
3. The conservatism corollary.
4. The developmental model.
5. The power of imitation.
6. The dynamics and relevance of social imagery.
7. The importance of social integration and participation.

may originate from early experience, as described earlier in the psychodynamic approach. Normalisation challenges carers to become acutely conscious of how their values, language and beliefs about people with a learning disability may adversely affect their care. For example, it is not uncommon for people to assume that people with a learning disability cannot form meaningful relationships resulting in marriage. The principles of normalisation challenge service providers to recognise that such a negative belief cannot, nor should not, be generalised to all people with a learning disability.

The relevance of role expectancy and role circularity. It is often found that people have low expectations of people with learning disabilities. This may serve to reinforce a person's disability because low expectation, in this context, results in reduced learning that in itself reinforces the nature of learning disability. Normalisation promotes positive role expectation by reinforcing the roles of people with a learning disability that will break the vicious circle of low expectation and therefore low performance.

The conservatism corollary. Chisholm (1993) described this core theme succinctly when he said 'conservatism corollary simply means that when a person has a characteristic which is not generally valued in society everything possible should be done to minimise that characteristic.' (Chisholm 1993). A concrete example of this core theme in action might be a carer encouraging a person with a learning disability, who persistently dribbles, to use a range of strategies to reduce the amount of dribbling for example, by attention to posture, breathing exercises and the use of tissues.

The developmental model. This core theme promotes the potential for growth and development in all individuals. It is clearly in keeping with the humanistic belief in self actualisation. To achieve such a core theme it would be important to ensure that all service-providing agencies made for adequate provision to meet the life-long learning needs of people with a learning disability.

The power of imitation. This theme acknowledges the importance of imitation or modelling to learning. Clearly during normal development much learning is achieved through imitating the behaviour of other significant people, for example brothers, sisters and friends. For the person with a learning disability there is no exception and it is imperative that good role models are available in a person's life so that they have adequate opportunities for learning.

The dynamics and relevance of social imagery. Learning disability has shouldered a negative imagery for many years. This theme acknowledges that this state of affairs must be tackled by identifying negative imagery and replacing it with positive imagery. There has been much work undertaken in this area by the Royal Society for Mentally Handicapped People.

The importance of social integration and participation. Finally, it is sometimes the case that people with a learning disability are segregated from others because of institutional care. It is imperative that these people are fully integrated and participate in community life beyond institutions. This serves to break the vicious cycle of stereotyping and labelling. Beacock (1992) believes that the humanist movement has made a significant impact upon the thinking of those charged with the responsibility for developing services for people with a learning disability. Since the 1970s there have been developments in the practicable implementation of normalisation and, in service provision the concept of normalisation has greatly affected the ways in which people with a learning disability are cared for. The principles of normalisation, when applied to service provision are both interesting and important. Chisholm (1993) said 'normalisation principles as a distinct entity have, to a greater or lesser extent, been applied in Britain since 1975 and the core value—that people with learning difficulties have the same human value as everyone else—is now written into virtually every service statement regarding planning and delivery of services in this country.' (Chisholm 1993). However, to achieve the ideal of 'the same rights and, wherever possible, the same responsibilities as others' has proved to be extremely problematic.

Activity 2.2 An exercise in the normalisation of people with learning disabilities

Identify three reasons why the ideals of normalisation might be difficult to achieve for a man with profound learning disability.

Although these core themes have been applied to learning disability, it is not inappropriate to apply them to other groups of people who may be devalued for example, the older person or those with mental health problems.

CONCLUSION

This chapter has put human beings centre stage in the study of the nature of communication, i.e. what and how do people communicate? We have seen that different models of the person rest on different underlying assumptions. Readers will, we hope, now be in a better position to reflect on their own assumptions about people when communicating with them and will be concious of the choices available from sources other than their own experiences. It is a basic theme of this book that with understanding and awareness it is possible to be more intentional, and hence more effective, in one's communication with others. We now turn to the wider social context in which human contact takes place to investigate its influence on communication.

REFERENCES

Atkinson R L, Atkinson R C, Smith E E, Bem D J, Hilgard E R 1990 Introduction to psychology, 10th edn. Harcourt Brace Jovanovich, London.
Balint M 1964 The doctor, his patient and the illness, 2nd edn. Tavistock/Routledge, London.
Beacock C 1992 Triggers for change. In: Thompson T, Mathias P 1992 Standards and mental handicap: keys to competence. Baillaire & Tindall, London.
Bellack A, Hersen M, Kazdin A 1982 International handbook of behaviour modification and therapy. Plenum Press, New York.
Chisholm A 1993 Quality of care. In: Shanley E, Stars T A Learning disabilities: a handbook of care, 2nd edn. Churchill, Edinburgh.
DOH 1992 Services for people with learning disabilities, challenging behaviour or mental health needs. HMSO, London.
Grunewald K 1969 The mentally retarded in Sweden. In: Recent advances in the study of subnormality, 2nd. edn. National Association for Mental Retardation, London.
Jones R, Connell E 1993 Ten years of gentle teaching: much ado about nothing? The Psychologist, Dec. 544-548.
Klein M 1963 Our adult world and its roots in infancy. Pitman, London.
Maslow A 1954 Motivation and personality. Harper and Row, New York.

McCue M 1993 Helping with behavioural problems. In: Shanley E, Stars T A Learning disabilities: a handbook of care, 2nd edn. Churchill, Edinburgh.
Menolascino F J and McGee J J 1991 Beyond gentle teaching: a non-aversive approach to helping those in need. Plenum Press, New York.
Noonan E 1983 Counselling young people. Methuen, London
Paul G, Bernstein D 1976 Anxiety and clinical problems: systematic desensitisation and related techniques. In: Spence J, Carson R, Thibaut 1976 Behavioural approaches to therapy. General Learning Press, New Jersey.
Pavlov I 1902 The work of the digestive glands. Trans. W H Thompson. Charles Griffin, London.
Pervin L A 1993 Personality: theory and research, 6th edn. John Wiley, New York.
Rogers C R 1970 On becoming a person: a therapist's view of psychotherapy. Houghton Mifflin, Boston.
Rogers C R 1974 On becoming a person, 4th edn. Constable, London
Skinner B F 1938 The behaviour of organisms. Appleton-Century Crofts, New York.
Watson J B 1924 Behaviourism (revised edition,1930). In: Stevanson L 1974 Seven theories of human nature. Oxford University Press, Oxford.
Wolfensberger W 1972 Normalisation. National Institute of Mental Retardation, Toronto.

FURTHER READING

Freud A 1986 The ego and the mechanisms of defence. Hogarth Press, London.
Medcof J & Roth L (eds) 1979 Approaches to psychology. Oxford University Press, Milton Keynes.
Ruddock R (ed) 1972 Six appraoches to the person. Routledge, London.

Stevenson L 1981 The study of human nature. Oxford University Press, Oxford.
Winnicott D W 1988 Human nature. Free Association Books, London.

Emphasis on practice

SECTION CONTENTS

3

Social factors affecting communication

Peter Morrall

THE SOCIAL CONTEXT

Drawing upon theory and research from sociology, social psychology, and anthropology, this chapter seeks to provide a number of insights into the complex social effects on interpersonal communication.

Communicating with other humans is considerably more complicated than it may at first seem. There are the obvious problems in understanding the explicit words and non-verbal behaviour, as well as the implicit messages that are being used by the people involved. However, apart from these interpersonal factors, communication is linked to the social environment in which it is taking place, and is effected by the social identity of those who are are participating (Figure 3.1).

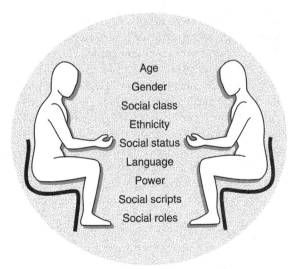

Figure 3.1 Social factors influencing interpersonal communication

All forms of communication start and end with individuals relaying or accepting messages. However, these messages are mediated by many other influences that cannot be comprehended fully (if at all) without reflecting upon both the immediate and the wider social context (McQuail 1984, Hartley 1993).

When a student nurse commences a new clinical experience, and introduces herself to a patient whom she has never met before, both are sending and receiving important signals about each other's social identity. Signals of identity, such as respective ages, gender, ethnic grouping, and status in society may influence the type of communication that takes place. Each identifies the other in a particular role, the student identifying the other person in the role of 'patient', and the patient perceiving the student in the role of 'nurse'.

Communication between professional colleagues will involve the same process of recognising each other's social attributes. Although age and gender still affect the form that the communication will take, what predominates at work is the prestige, power, and control that each nurse is ascribed by the organisation (and ultimately by society).

Hancock states that the '...way in which we respond to a communication will often depend upon the status of the person making it. A statement from the Prime Minister will be given more weight than one from Mr. Jones next door...The Prime Minister might say something utterly banal, but we would still tend to listen to what he had to say...' (Hancock, 1971, p.63).

Interactions between a student nurse and a consultant surgeon will be shaped significantly by the relatively low status of the former and the relatively high status of the latter.

Activity 3.1 An exercise in social identity

Examine your reactions to the next three people you meet. Apart from what was stated verbally, what 'hidden' messages were being transmitted by you and by them about your respective status, age, social class, gender etc.?

Habermas (1976) observed in the case of politicians (who he believes are not held in the

high esteem they once were) that the status given to a particular role may rise or fall. With respect to nurses and doctors, it could be argued that certain government policies, such as the introduction of general management into the health service, will result in a narrowing of the difference in status between the two professional groups.

This chapter makes the point that whatever and however people communicate it is not done in a neutral way. Messages sent verbally or non-verbally are moderated to comply with the norms of the society to which we belong. The communication that occurs at an interpersonal level is not conducted in a social vacuum. Nurses need to reflect upon the social context in which a communication takes place to fully understand what it implies.

FREE WILL AND SOCIAL INFLUENCE

Social considerations may dictate the content, style and outcome of the communication that occurs between individuals. Similarly, the conversational interaction between a nurse and a service user or a professional colleague may be pre-organised by each participant's gender identity, age, ethnic origin, educational background, and overall status in society.

An 18-year-old student nurse and a 60-year-old company director who is in hospital with a myocardial infarction, may find it hard to ignore the social attributes, experience, and particular world view that each has and to have an interchange of opinions. Can they talk to each other without their words being shaped and limited by the difference in their age, and social status?

Hartley comments that there is '...something of a battle...between those who regard society as the backdrop against which humans choose to act and those who feel that society creates or determines the ways in which we act' (op. cit., p. 80).

The sociologist Giddens (1984) has attempted to show that human behaviour is not totally under the control of the individual, nor is it completely shaped by society. Giddens tries to bridge the gap between those theorists who believe that people act voluntarily, i.e. they have free choice over what they do, and those theorists who argue that human behaviour is completely determined by society.

It is the synthesis of the two extremes of voluntarism and determinism, as advocated by Giddens, that may be the most appropriate theoretical approach to understanding inter-personal communication. That is, humans do have choice in what they think, do and say, but this is constrained in varying degrees by social factors. The nurse's interaction with service users and colleagues will be controlled in part by the personal attributes of all of those concerned, e.g. their attitudes, personality and intellect, as well as by such socially prescribed attributes as 'role' and 'status'.

The individual therefore belongs to a society which has a pre-given structure. Rules, written laws, roles and relationships make up the structure and unwritten regulations determine what is acceptable and what is unacceptable behaviour.

The structure exists only in the abstract sense, but provides a framework which supports and regulates all human activities.

Power and status

Hogg and Abrams (1988) believe that 'power' and 'status' characterise the structure of a society. They suggest that people can be divided into numerous categories on the basis of such social traits as gender, religion, occupation, nationality and class. For Hogg and Abrams, these social categories have different amounts of influence and prestige.

An individual who is unemployed is in a different 'structural' position in society to another individual employed as a lawyer. The former has little power and status, the latter has a considerable amount of both. Although these structural elements regulate human behaviour to a significant degree, individual human action influences the structure of society. A male hospital manager in conversation with a female staff nurse on a medical ward may have more power allocated to him because of gender identity and work-related role. Therefore, he is more likely

to achieve his goal of reducing costs than the staff nurse who seeks an increase in resources. Nevertheless, the staff nurse has some potential influence. At one level she may have access to information, e.g. about the quality of care in her clinical area, that enables her to negotiate rather than just accept the manager's viewpoint. At another level, the staff nurse may join a political movement which aims to put pressure on the government to provide more funds for the National Health Service.

Whether the concept of society is that of a set of structures that shapes all behaviour; or nothing more than the accumulation of actions and thoughts that occur between individuals, there is a common emphasis on communication. The structure of society and interpersonal comm-unication, together with other systems of communication, such as the mass media, are linked reflexively. What people say to each other will help shape the structures in society, and these structures in society will, in turn, influence communications.

Humans have choice in what and how they communicate, but this is moderated by social structures.

Activity 3.2   Social influences on communication

List ten forms of communication that exist in society. Describe the ways in which you influence these forms of communication, and the ways in which they influence you.

SCRIPTS AND ROLES

One way of trying to comprehend the effects of the social context on communication is to view all interaction between human beings as representing a stage-play or drama. That is, what we say and do to each other is part of a scripted performance. Each actor performs one or many roles during a performance. Tajfel & Fraser (1978) believe 'role is the required behaviour of someone in a given position...the term "role performance" refers to the actual behaviour of the incumbent' (Tajfel and Fraser, 1978).

Entering into a clinical situation is similar to being an actor in a play, where service users, doctors and nurses are the actors in the cast. When interacting with a patient, communications are organised through the medium of the social role of a 'nurse' and communications are affected by the socially prescribed expectations of that role. Equally, the patient is communicating through her socially prescribed identity as a 'patient'.

Examples of the roles that may be enacted during any one day include possibly that of student nurse, son or daughter, brother or sister, friend and member of a sports team (Figure 3.2). Each role serves as a social template which fashions both what is sent by the communicator and what is received by the other person. However, the way people behave in these roles will depend partly on how others behave towards them. If a student nurse is treated as subservient to doctors and senior nurses then the script will be different to that followed when she is treated as an adult by her personal tutor.

To follow the rules of a particular role, people need to know how others in associated roles behave. Hospital patients require information about the performances of the 'actors' they are going to meet in the hospital setting, e.g. the nurses, doctors, physiotherapists, ward clerks and domestics. For any role to exist, others must be performing in their roles. An individual cannot be a student nurse unless there are qualified nurses, nurse lecturers, and patients!

This theory of 'dramaturgy' has been advanced by, amongst others, Erving Goffman (1959). What Goffman proposed was that scripts serve as guidelines which, through experience and the process of socialisation, enable people to know how to behave in different circumstances.

Activity 3.3 An exercise in social roles

Describe the social roles that you have performed in the last week. What are the differences between how others might have expected you to perform in these roles and how you actually performed?

RULES AND CONFLICT

Guidelines for social behaviour are regulated by specific rules that apply to the individual's particular circumstances. These rules predict how nurses will act when they are in the lecture theatre, on the ward, or at a dance.

Problems arise when an individual enters a new situation and doesn't know the rules. However, general patterns of behaviour from previous experiences will suggest what actions might be normal and acceptable.

Student nurses may have faced, and be expected to face continuously, many novel and anxiety-provoking situations, for example, the first day in college or a new clinical experience. It may be considered important to get the rules of communication right in all social situations and particularly when meeting lecturers, other students, or colleagues for the first time. There will be a constant search for the right thing to say and the appropriate gestures to make, combined with the recognition of social space and the necessary use of eye contact.

Getting it wrong can cause lasting embarrassment. That is why some individuals try not to communicate too much, either verbally or non-verbally, until they have discovered what the rules are.

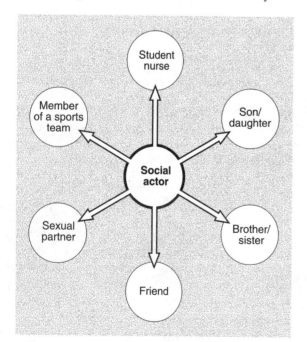

Figure 3.2 Examples of a social actor's multiple roles

Activity 3.4   The influence of social rules on behaviour

Reflect upon your own behaviour, and that of service users, when entering into new situations.

How do we discover what is appropriate, and what is not appropriate, to say and do in these situations?

Just as student nurses have to sort out what to do in new situations, service users entering into hospital as in-patients or out-patients have to establish what the appropriate behaviour is in their role as patient. They have to find out what the organisational and interpersonal rules are, and this adds to the concerns they will already have for their clinical condition. A service user who is told that she has a major illness or disability may have to reconstitute many of her former role behaviours. Someone who has to have a leg amputated may not be able to perform her previous role at work or leisure.

In practice, roles cannot easily be compartmentalised as they have elaborate interconnections with each other. Some of the behaviour demonstrated in the role of friend may be replicated in the role of nurse. Although some of the behaviour expected in one role may be complementary to another there may be circumstances when roles are in tension. Abraham & Shanley (1992) explained

As we move from one situation to another we may occupy the roles of nurse, club secretary, team member, mother, daughter, and political campaigner...The demands of these roles compete for our time and energy, leading to role conflict. A typical source of such role conflict is between obligations to family members and to those at work.

(Abraham & Shanley, 1992)

In addition to the conflict arising when the expectations of the different roles are incompatible, there are a number of other types of role conflict (Hargreaves, 1972; Tajfel & Fraser, op.cit.). For example, there may be disagreement amongst role occupants about the content of the role. Student nurses may have different views about what their role should be; some may study harder than others; some may view their role as 'just a job', whereas others may feel that nursing is a vocation (Mackay 1990). Individuals in other associated roles may disagree with the role

occupant's interpretation of how to perform that role. Senior nurses perhaps have views about the way in which student nurses communicate with patients and other staff. These could be different to the views of the students themselves (Stockwell 1972).

Role conflict is managed through a number of different strategies. One example is where individuals distance themselves from one or more of their roles. Nursing may still be regarded as a female occupation. Therefore, the conflict between the gender and occupational identity of a male student nurse may be diffused by the nurse joking about his role, or by stating that he intends to eventually become an educationalist or a manager.

THE SICK ROLE AND COMPLIANCE

Being ill may be regarded as performing a role just as more intentional roles are performed. Biological or psychological changes may cause illness, but according to social theorists, such as Parsons (1951), there is a type of socially acceptable behaviour for people who are ill. Parsons argues that illness itself is a form of deviant behaviour which has to be regulated in order that society can continue to operate effectively. Too much uncontrolled illness in society would lead to problems at work and the smooth running of industry would be disrupted.

The sick role can be regarded as a 'contract' between the person who is ill and the rest of society, the latter being represented by the health care professions. These professions control access to the sick role. When an individual enters the sick role she is given a number of privileges by society, but also has a number of obligations to society. The sick person is exempt from work and family responsibilities, and is not blamed for being ill. However, she must seek and follow medical advice, and must want to recover as quickly as possible.

There is much debate about how realistic Parson's concept of the sick role is in today's society (Turner 1987 Ch. 3; Gerhardt 1987). With reference to interpersonal communication, the concept does point to a social pressure on patients to perform in a particular way once they have accepted the role of being sick. If patients want to be regarded as having a legitimate illness they are encouraged to accept the treatment offered by those involved in their care. As a consequence of an individual entering into the sick role, with its concomitant obligations and rights, verbal and non-verbal behaviour would tend to be passive and compliant.

Activity 3.5   Attitudes towards the 'sick role'

Describe how your verbal and non-verbal behaviour (or that of your friends and members of your family) alters once the role of being sick has been accepted. Are there any differences between the sick role behaviour of men compared to that of women?

Non-compliance

Although a patient may appear to accept what doctors, nurses, and other health care professionals suggest, the eventual outcome may be a modification or rejection of the treatment or advice by the patient. Patients may not turn up for appointments, they may ignore medications as prescribed, and they may reject health education recommendations, such as giving up smoking, taking more exercise and reducing intake of alcohol.

The disparity between what appears to be happening and what actually is happening may also be true in the doctor/nurse relationship (Stein 1968). He suggests that a 'game' is being played between doctors and nurses. Nurses appear to comply with the instructions given by doctors in that there is very little open conflict, but nurses find indirect ways of communicating their opinions and gaining influence about the care and treatment of patients. These indirect manoeuvres are recognised by doctors, but nurses can still 'get their own way' because they do not directly challenge the authority of the doctor. What is at issue is not whose opinion is accepted, but that the hierarchical structure remains unaffected.

In doctor/patient relationships, non-compliance can increase when the patient is not offered the opportunity to participate in the

conversation between herself and the medical practitioner. It can also increase when the patient is given little information about her condition (Hauser 1981; Morgan et al 1985).

The use of professional jargon is another effective verbal method of control. Patients will probably not understand what is being said, and this will lead to a perception of the doctor as the 'expert' and themselves as the novice.

Control is exercised not only through verbal or 'informational' strategies, but also through organisational settings and non-verbal signals. If the patient is in hospital she is on unfamiliar territory which means that she is more likely to be influenced by the health care professional. If the health care professional visits the patient in her own home then to some extent the balance of power shifts in favour of the patient. Non-verbal cues from the professional, together with the physical environment can either intimidate the patient, or provide encouragement for her to participate more actively. Morgan (1991) stated:

By looking interested, nodding encouragingly and other gestures doctors can provide positive feedback to patients, whereas by continued rifling through notes, twiddling with pens, or failing to look directly at patients, they may convey disinterest...Interaction is also influenced by the seating and relative positions of doctor and patient....

(Morgan, 1991, p.60)

Morgan (ibid.) points out that the health care professional may use clinical procedures as an effective way of controlling the interaction. Whilst the nurse or doctor is concentrating on what would appear to be an important clinical technique, the patient is potentially silenced.

There is evidence that conversations between nurses and patients tend to be oriented towards nursing tasks rather than acknowledging the patient's anxieties and her views (Faulkner 1979; Macleod Clark 1981; Melia 1987). This lack of empathic appreciation of the patient's experience of her clinical condition and of the service being offered by the health system may result in ineffective service delivery. This may comprise uninvestigated non-compliance, perception of patients as 'lost causes' and an increased likelihood of mistaken diagnosis and treatment recommendations (Abraham & Shanley, op. cit.)

The balance of control over what happens between health care professionals in face-to-face interaction may start to shift more in the patient's favour with the trend for service users to become better informed about medical practices and more empowered as consumers (Salvage 1992).

POWER

Very much linked to the notion of control is the concept of power. For an individual or group to gain control there must be some degree of power available to them. Power exists when an individual behaves in such a way that it will produce a change in another individual (Cartwright & Zander 1968). A nurse who explains the ward routine to a patient has the power to reduce the patient's anxiety about being in hospital. The community nurse who demonstrates to the patient how to self-medicate has the power to reduce the patient's reliance on the nurse.

A number of different sources of power have been identified in Box 3.1 (French & Raven 1959, Collins & Raven 1969).

McQuail (op. cit.) indicates a number of generalisations that may be made about the ways in which power can be exploited through communication:

- Monopolising the conversation can have the effect of gaining control and achieving a desired outcome. Where dominance occurs, and goes unchallenged, the greater the influence.
- A person can ensure a message is accepted by making it coincide with the beliefs of the other person. The content of the message will also be important in determining how influential the communicator will be. For example, the influence will be greater if the topic under discussion is about an issue with which the other person has no personal experience.
- Someone who is regarded as credible and having high status, through being physically attractive, intellectually admired and with much in common with the audience, will be far more powerful than someone who has less attractive attributes.

Box 3.1	Sources of power
1. Expert power:	where it is assumed that someone has greater knowledge and skills than others because of their long training or experience (e.g. as in the doctor/patient or lecturer/student relationship).
2. Coercive power:	where an individual can control the punishment of another (e.g. a parent deciding to smack her child).
3 Reward power:	where an individual has the ability to reward another either by providing positive elements or by removing negative ones (e.g. as in some forms of treatment programmes for people with learning difficulties who are given praise when they learn a new skill).
4. Legitimate power:	where it is accepted that a person has the right and authority of society to have influence over others (e.g. a judge, police officer, or the 'nurse in charge' of the clinical treatment).
5. Referent power:	where one person has attributes that others wish they had and try to identify with (e.g. an individual may try to emulate a particular colleague whom she admires).
6. Informational power:	when a person obtains information that others do not have, she demonstrates power by controlling how much of the information she is going to supply (e.g. as in the case of deciding whether or not to tell a patient that she is going to die). (French & Raven 1959; Collins & Raven 1969)

- Being a patient and a student nurse carries a relatively low amount of prestige in health care organisations compared to that received by the qualified health care professionals. Both the patient and the student nurse are in a different structural position to the qualified staff who are seen as permanent, whereas the patient and the student are transient. If either is also disliked and appears unattractive then it is very unlikely they will be listened to!
- Power is socially prescribed to a large degree. Society confers power on those in authority.

Sometimes power may be gained through the acquiesence of others. Indeed power can be removed from those who have it.

- At an interpersonal level, many patients are becoming more assertive in their dealings with medical personnel. Student nurses, because of the adoption of more student and adult-centred approaches to learning, might become less accepting of the traditional and hier-archical power-relationships found within health care institutions.

Activity 3.6   The use and exploitation of power in communication

Observe the ways in which you, other nurses, and doctors exercise power by controlling the content and style of what is communicated when in discussion with service users. What influence do the physical characteristics of the participants have on these occasions?

DISCOURSE

Acknowledging the existence of 'power' in social relationships suggests that communications are not always carried out on an equal basis. The objectives of those who have power in society and in interpersonal relationships are often achieved through manipulating or 'distorting' commun-ication (Malhotra 1987).

According to Jurgen Habermas (1970, 1972) what is communicated has the appearance of being understood, equitable and acceptable to each individual, but below the surface there may be a 'hidden agenda' which is directed by the person (or group) with power. Forms of communication, such as language, are organised to ensure an outcome that is in the interest of the powerful individual. It is indicative of the power of this individual that the communication process can be organised in this way.

From the health care arena, Hugman (1991) provides an example of power-distorted communication in Box 3.2.

People with power have the ability to select the content and style of what is being communicated. This is done through particular symbols,

---

Box 3.2   An example of power-distorted communication (Hugman, 1991)

A caring professional 'asks' a service user to comply with an intervention (to take medicine, do the exercises, take part in family therapy), but the request is directed to accomplishing the professional goals and not to reaching an agreement with the service user which gives the service user's goals an equal status in the relationship. (Hugman 1991, p.35.)

---

practices, and styles of language that ensure domination. The organising of communication on the basis of power is described as 'discourse'.

Many powerful factions in society develop their own discourse, including professional groups. The variety of discourse that health care professionals adopt has been studied by Michel Foucault (1971, 1973, 1974, 1980). In particular Foucault examined how medical knowledge has been constructed to form an apparently legitimate, and consequently influential, way of viewing the world. He points out that there cannot be one 'factual' way of viewing the world because different societies, both historically and cross-culturally, have different realities.

This line of reasoning would imply that seemingly real entities such as 'health' and 'disease' are not real at all.

Diabetes, obesity, anorexia nervosa, hyper-activity, heart disease and dementia are arbitrary categories whose existence, boundaries, and importance to society have changed in the past and will change in the future. The way in which service users think and talk about their bodies is controlled by the concepts, theories and symbols that have been supplied by health care profes-sionals.

The medical discourse in turn is a reflection of what those with power in society have deemed to be of significance at that point in time.

Asking patients about their exercise, smoking and drinking habits, and encouraging them to take more responsibility for their health is not simply an example of good medical and nursing practice. These things are being discussed because of social, economic and political contingencies that lie beyond the face-to-face encounter between service user and health care professional. They are the consequence of such historical processes as the Enlightenment and industrial-isation. Processes such as these gradually changed our attitudes about what was important in society from religion and 'the community' to a belief in the specialness and sanctity of the individual human being and the body (Brooks 1993).

Activity 3.7   Power-distorted communication

Gaining permission from those involved first, tape-record a discussion between a number of different health care professionals (perhaps at a multi-disciplinary meeting). Analyse the tape for power-distorted communications.

SOCIOLINGUISTICS

One important aspect of discourse is language. The discipline of sociolinguistics explores how social factors moderate language. Language, as with all other forms of communication, is not context-free. There is a direct link between the manner of speech, the words used and how society is structured.

Membership of social groupings provides people with a particular form of linguistic expression. The way a person speaks may provide the listener with an immediate clue as to her status in society and her membership of an identifiable group. Members of the Royal family have verbal mannerisms that differ from the majority of the population.

In societies where there are ethnic groupings, the way in which language is used can imply that the social status of the speaker may determine how others regard her.

Nurses are socialised to use a form of language that identifies them with other nurses and other health care professionals. They belong to a 'speech community' of nurses within which there is a sharing of verbal signs and professional jargon (Gumperz 1968). The use of the specialised language associated with health care will symbolise to colleagues group membership, and to others that they are excluded from that grouping (Miller & Form 1962).

One form of speech, such as technical jargon, may predominate when nurses are amongst other nurses. Professionals speak differently though when they are with different speech communities. When people are with their family they will use words, phrases and intonations that are appropriate to the shared meanings that have developed in that social group rather than those they have learned in their professional role.

Activity 3.8   An exercise in sociolinguistics

List ten words or phrases that nurses use exclusively. What are the effects of using exclusive language on others (e.g. service users)?

LANGUAGE AND SOCIAL CLASS

The very nature of the health system in Britain means that nurses communicate with service users and colleagues from diverse social class backgrounds. Members of different social classes have separate ways of expressing themselves.

Most people acknowledge the existence of some form of class structure. Social theorists, however, are not able to agree about the criteria for distinguishing the various social class groupings (Worsley 1987). Some believe that traditional class boundaries are in the process of disintegration (Crook et al 1992).

Whatever criteria are used to define social class, it would appear to influence language. Research by Schatzman & Strauss (1954) in America indicated that there were significant variations between working and middle class use of language. The people who were designated as working class in the study talked of experiences with which they were familiar but the listener was not. They would not, however, attempt to 'clue in' the listener by giving background information. On the other hand, the middle class participants did help the listener to understand by supplying extra details.

In Britain, research by Bernstein (1975) has indicated a strong link between the social class to which an individual belongs and the form of speech in use. Bernstein argued that working class people use a different linguistic code to that used by middle class people. The former utilise a restricted, or context-tied code whereas the latter make use of an elaborated code.

The restricted code is simpler, involves short, sharp exchanges, deals with practical matters, and is tied to the immediate context of the conversation. The meaning of the communications with this code is often implicit. There is the assumption that the listener will know what is being talked about and little effort is made to provide what might appear to the speaker to be superfluous description. As the term implies, the elaborated code is more explanatory, complex, and abstract. With the elaborated code there is a more explicit verbalisation of the meanings that the user of the restricted code takes for granted.

Critics of Bernstein's work have challenged his view that the restricted code is simpler than the elaborated code, and the implication that it is in some way inferior (Labov 1978). It is suggested that the language of the working class is as subtle as that of the middle class, but with different grammatical rules.

Furthermore, individuals may adopt both types of code depending on the circumstances. When two old friends meet, who have known each other since childhood, they use a restricted code because certain gestures or phrases 'speak a thousand words'. But when each is in a more formal environment they will use the elaborated code because of the need to explain concepts and ideas to unfamiliar people.

Activity 3.9   The use of linguistic codes

Describe the type of linguistic code used by you, your friends, your peers, and other health care professionals you come into contact with. Do you change your code depending upon with whom you are communicating?

LANGUAGE AND GENDER

Individuals are genetically endowed with male or female physical characteristics, but how they behave as men and women is largely socially prescribed.

Studies of male and female behaviour in divergent cultural settings provide evidence to suggest that, to a significant extent, being a man or a woman is a social role. This view is supported by many anthropological studies of pre-industrial, industrial, and post-industrial societies. As Helman (1990) reports, researchers have discovered a great variety of behaviour classified as appropriate for men and women.

Every society has its own set of acceptable patterns of behaviour or norms for the role of male and female. Language often demonstrates what is considered to be 'natural' behaviour for these roles. Lakoff (1975) discovered that in conversation men tended to be direct and assertive, whereas women were overpolite and passive.

In many western societies the expected different role behaviours of the two genders is not as it was in the past. Women wear trousers, men wear ear-rings, women go out to work, and men train to be nurses.

As Hogg & Abrams (op. cit.) note, there have also been changes in the more obvious ways in which language is used to differentiate between the two genders. Chairmen are now chairpersons, mankind has been renamed humanity and househusbands exist alongside housewives. Whether these changes are substantial or superficial remains questionable. Expectations of what is considered to be an appropriate way of behaving for a man or for a woman may not have altered fundamentally.

Tannen (1992) argues that men and women actually speak different dialects, which she terms 'genderlects'. She suggests that communication between men and women is as hampered as communication would be between two people from different cultures.

The genderlect of men is based on notions of independence and status, whereas that of women is based on connection and intimacy.

Men's talk frequently involves overt and covert references to the importance in personal and working relationships of maintaining their freedom to choose what they want to do, and of achieving high prestige. On the other hand, women regard it of greater importance to formulate close personal alliances with colleagues, family, and friends. Tannen observes, however, that in situations where men and women are together in mixed-gender team meetings or classrooms, the male genderlect tends to dominate as this is perceived to be the norm by both men and women.

The research into gender and language has important implications for the way in which nurses communicate with service users and other health care professionals. There is the suggestion that female nurses 'miscommunicate' with male patients, and male nurses 'miscommunicate' with female patients. Consequently, in these circumstances the needs of service users are not even understood, let alone met!

The majority of nurses are women, and therefore the occupation of nursing has a communicative bias towards a female genderlect. This, however, may serve to prohibit the full professional emancipation of nursing. Whilst nursing communicates passivity, connection and intimacy, the male-dominated profession of medicine may maintain its superior position in the hierarchy of health care professions by communicating assertively its own high esteem, and the right to be autonomous in clinical practice.

Activity 3.10   An exercise in the use of genderlects

Examine male and female speech (e.g. by using a tape-recorder). Can you identify competing genderlects? If so, what are the characteristics of these genderlects?

CONCLUSION

Nurses are in an occupation that has interpersonal communication at its core. Virtually all nursing work revolves around the need for nurses to be effective communicators, whether relating to colleagues or with service users. This is indicated in the content of contemporary educational programmes.

Although the subject of interpersonal communication now receives considerable attention from nurse educators, it is of little value to examine communication at the level of the overt verbal and non-verbal messages.

When reflecting upon acts of interpersonal communication there is a requirement to consider the wider social context, the social characteristics of the sender and receiver of the communication, and the structure of the power relationships between those involved. There is a necessity for nurses to become sensitive to how their communications are influenced and distorted by social factors before accurate communication, or what Habermas (op. cit.) describes as 'communicative competency', can be achieved.

REFERENCES

Abraham C, Shanley E 1992 Social psychology for nurses. Edward Arnold, London.
Bernstein B 1975 Class, codes and control. Routledge & Kegan Paul, London.
Brooks P 1993 Body works: objects of desire in modern narrative. Harvard University Press, Harvard.
Cartwright D, Zander A (eds) 1968 Group dynamics, 3rd edn. Tavistock, London.
Collins B E, Raven B H 1969 Group structure: attraction, coalitions, communication and power. In: Lindzey G, Aronson E (eds) The handbook of social psychology, Vol.4, 2nd edn. Addison-Wesley, Reading, Mass.
Crook S, Pakulski J, Waters M 1992 Postmodernisation: change in advanced society. Sage, London.
Faulkner A 1979 Monitoring nurse/patient conversations in the ward. Nursing Times, 75, Supplement, 95-96.
Foucault M 1971 Madness and civilisation. Tavistock, London.
Foucault M 1973 The birth of the clinic. Tavistock, London.
Foucault M 1974 The order of things. Tavistock, London.
Foucault M 1980 Power/knowledge, selected interviews and other writings 1972-1977. Harvester, Brighton.
French J R P, Raven B H 1959 The bases of social power. In: Cartwright D (ed.) Studies in social power. University of Michigan Press, Michigan.

Gerhardt U 1987 Parson's role theory and health interaction. In: Scambler G (ed) Sociological theory and medical sociology. Tavistock, London.
Giddens A 1984 The constitution of society. Polity Press, Cambridge.
Goffman E 1959 The presentation of self in everyday life. Penguin, Harmondsworth.
Gumperz J 1968 The speech community. International encyclopedia of the social sciences, 2nd edn. Macmillan, London.
Habermas J 1970 Towards a rational society. Heinemann, London.
Habermas J 1972 Knowledge and human interests. Heinemann, London.
Habermas J 1976 Legitimation crisis. Beacon, Boston.
Hancock A 1971 Communication. Heinemann, London.
Hargreaves D 1972 Interpersonal relations and education. Routledge & Kegan Paul, London.
Hartley P 1993 Interpersonal communication. Routledge, London.
Hauser S T 1981 Physician/patient relationships. In: Mishler E G, Amaraingham L R, Osherson S D, Hauser S T, Waxler N E, Liem R (eds) Social contexts of health, illness and patient care. Cambridge University Press, Cambridge.

Helman C G 1990 Culture, health and illness, 2nd edn. Wright, London.

Hogg M A, Abrams D 1988 Social identifications. Routledge, London.

Hugman R 1991 Power in caring professions. Macmillan, Basingstoke.

Labov W 1978 Sociolinguistic patterns. Blackwell, Oxford.

Lakoff R 1975 Language and a woman's place. Harper and Row, New York.

Mackay L 1990 Nursing: just another job? In: Abbott P, Wallace W (eds) The sociology of the caring professions. Falmer, London.

Macleod Clark J 1981 Communication in nursing. Nursing Times, 1 January, 12-18.

McQuail D 1984 Communication, 2nd edn. Longman, Harlow.

Malhotra V A 1987 Habermas' sociological theory as a basis for clinical practice with small groups. Clinical Sociology Review, 5, 181-192.

Melia K 1987 Learning and working: the occupational socialisation of nurses. Tavistock, London.

Miller D C, Form W H 1962 Industrial sociology. Harper and Row, London.

Morgan M 1991 The doctor/patient relationship. In: Scambler G (ed) Sociology as applied to medicine, 3rd edn. Baillere Tindall, London.

Morgan M, Calnan M, Manning N 1985 Sociological approaches to health and medicine. Croom Helm, London.

Parsons T 1951 The social system. Rouledge & Kegan Paul, London.

Salvage J 1992 The new nursing: empowering patients or empowering nurses? In: Robinson J, Gray A, Elkan R (eds) Policy issues in nursing. Open University Press, Milton Keynes.

Schatzman L, Strauss A 1954 Social class and modes of communication. American Journal of Sociology. 60, 329-38.

Stein L I 1968 The doctor/nurse game. American Journal of Nursing. 68, 1-5.

Stockwell F 1972 The unpopular patient: the study of nursing care reports. Series 1, No.2. Royal College of Nursing, London.

Tajfel H, Fraser C 1978 Introducing social psychology. Penguin, Harmondsworth.

Tannen D 1992 You just don't understand: women and men in conversation. Virago, London.

Turner B S 1987 Medical power and social knowledge. Sage, London.

Worsley P 1987 The new introducing sociology. Penguin, Harmondsworth.

FURTHER READING

Atkinson P 1990 The ethnographic imagination: textual constructions of reality. Routledge, London.

Social Trends 1992. HMSO, London.

4

Psychological factors affecting communication

Stuart A. Hindle

INTRODUCTION

In Chapter 1, the differences between inter- and intrapersonal communication were described. In practice, they interact with each other in subtle ways.

This chapter will explore those differences and introduce the concept of communication filters and the ways in which context influences communication.

THE INTER / INTRAPERSONAL MIX

Human communication is a highly complex activity of interaction involving others as well as oneself. What one person intends in the interaction is not always understood by the other person. Consider the example given in Box 4.1.

Box 4.1   The interaction of inter- and intrapersonal factors

---

Sarah Jones arrived for her first day on the Project 2000 nursing course. She was anxious about meeting new people and her bladder was feeling full. She had expectations of the course tutors that were based on her perceptions of teachers from her school days.

The other students looked so bright and confident, Sarah was sure they would have no trouble on the course. The tutors introduced themselves and gave a brief talk about the course: its structure, the assessment strategy and the competencies to be achieved.

After 30 minutes, the tutors felt satisfied that they had introduced themselves and given an overview of the course. Sarah on the other hand was confused—she did not yet know any of the other students and felt her bladder was about to burst.

Box 4.1 shows how, on the surface, it would seem that information had been given from one person to another in a quiet room with no apparent distractions. The Oxford Dictionary describes communication as 'something that communicates information from one person to another'. However, this does not take account of the complex interpersonal and extrapersonal factors that are involved.

In the example given in Box 4.1, Sarah was anxious about meeting new people in a new setting and her bladder was becoming increasingly uncomfortable. The terms used by tutors to describe the course were unfamiliar to Sarah, and were forgotten almost immediately. There were certain communication filters involved that blocked or distorted the message sent from the tutors. These filters will be discussed in detail later in the chapter, but briefly they consist of :

- Defence mechanisms
- Beliefs and values
- Assumptions
- Prejudices
- Perceptual distortions

Several authors have attempted to devise a model of the intrapersonal factors involved in communication episodes (Pluckman 1978, Hargie & Marshall 1986). These are summarised in Figure 4. 1.

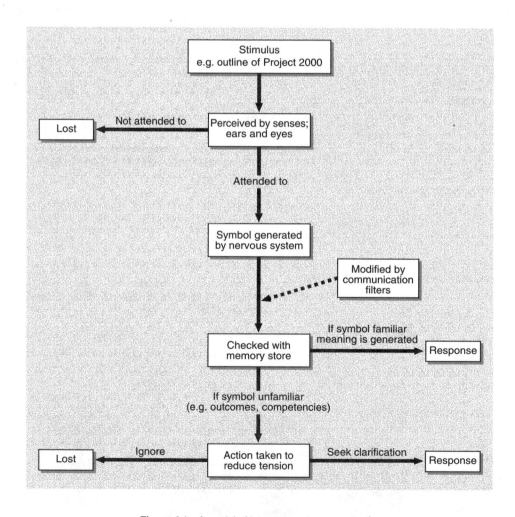

Figure 4.1 A model of intrapersonal communication

In this process, the sense organs receive stimuli. The nervous system then perceives these stimuli, processing them into symbols that are then checked with those already stored in the memory. This is the point at which all a person's past experiences, attitudes, beliefs and values influence what happens next. If there is consistency between what is perceived and all these factors, then meaning is generated and a response occurs. However, if as in Sarah's case, there is an incongruity because of her lack of understanding and an overriding need to find the toilet, then meaning will be lost.

Maslow (1954) pointed out in his human needs hierarchy, that unless basic physiological needs are met (including the need to empty the bladder) little else will be of importance. In the example given, had tutorial staff offered beverages before the introduction, pointed out where the toilets were, and asked for any questions, the intrapersonal conflict that occurred could have been at least partially resolved. Tutorial staff had obviously been through the process of introducing students to the course on several occasions and because they were no longer sensitive to the technical language, they assumed that the students had the same level of understanding.

Unfortunately this is a trap into which many professionals fall. Medical and nursing staff become so accustomed to using technical language with each other that when they give information to patients, it too becomes loaded with jargon. It is important, therefore, for nurses to communicate with patients at an appropriate level of understanding, as outlined in Chapter 5.

METACOMMUNICATIONS

There are two aspects to communication, verbal and non-verbal. Occasionally, there are incongruencies between the verbal and the non-verbal message, as when someone who is asked how they are feeling, replies 'alright' yet shrugs his shoulders and looks away.

The verbal message is 'I'm feeling fine' but the non-verbal message is 'I'm not really'.

Another example is the crossing of fingers behind one's back when telling a lie. Here, the non-verbal message would not be as obvious to a second person.

In this second example, the behaviour is referring to communication itself. This is known as metacommunication. In verbal communication, there are two types of message—content and relational.

Content messages, according to Adler & Rodman (1991), are those which are about the topic under discussion. For example 'It's your turn to empty the dustbin' is an obvious content message. However, this same statement can have a relational component to it. Relational messages convey how one person feels towards another.

Try the following activity.

Activity 4.1 Content and relational messages

Think of two ways of saying 'It's your turn to empty the dustbin', one that is demanding and the other that is matter-of-fact. Notice how the non-verbal message is conveyed in each example.

Try this with other examples of content messages.

To summarise, content messages are obvious and are verbal, whereas relational messages are usually non-verbal and therefore less explicit. It is suggested that 60% of communication is non-verbal and can be ambiguous.

It is a good idea to check one's perception of a verbal interaction in case the wrong assumption has been made. In the previous example, if the request to empty the dustbin had been made in a demanding tone of voice, this could be checked by saying 'When you use that tone of voice, I get the idea that you are angry with me. Is that right?' If the other person was going through a particularly stressful time, it could be that he hadn't realised that he came across in such a demanding way, and a potential conflict could be avoided.

This perceptual check is an example of the verbal form of a relational message; a communication about communication or metacommunication.

Any discussions about relationships are metacommunicational and are very useful in keeping a relationship honest and constructive. It provides a way of solving conflicts in a constructive way, by moving the emphasis from content to relational issues.

Imagine a man and woman arguing over going out to the pub, one wanting to go and the other wanting to stay in for the evening. It may be that the argument is relational. For example, one partner could say 'It's not that I want to go out and you don't that's the problem. I think it's that you're mad with me because I go out with the lads three nights a week. Is that how you are feeling?' Of course, this may not be the case, but at least the other person can confirm or deny it and progress can be made in communicating with one another.

As with all communication skills, meta-communication has to be used appropriately. If overused, the other person might think they were being constantly analysed.

Another area where metacommunication could be appropriate is in the giving of compliments. This is a sadly neglected area especially in the workplace. If someone is paid a compliment about the way in which they talk to patients, it is likely they will feel appreciated and persist with the behaviour in future.

INCONGRUENCIES IN RECEIVED MESSAGES

If having checked a person's behaviour by using a relational statement, the person flatly denies the emotion yet non-verbally is obviously sending that message through facial expression, gestures or posture, then there is a mismatch between what appears obvious non-verbally and what the person is saying. This is an incongruity and could be due to one of the following reasons:

1. Falseness or deceit as described by Carl Rogers (1961) where the person is consciously attempting to deny the emotion. An example could be when a student nurse observes a staff nurse carrying out a procedure which she feels is out of date, but does not want to show her feelings and will not express them.
2. Denial, where the response is unconsciously motivated. Denial is one of the defence mechanisms described later in this chapter

Whilst a person can be very good at controlling verbal communication when attempting to deceive others, non-verbal behaviour is less easy to hide. Facial expression and posture can be manipulated to fit in with the verbal message to some extent, but movements of the legs, feet and hands, can give away incongruity or insincerity. The reasons why individuals may act insincerely is because of a wish to be accepted by others, not to rock the boat or to be laughed at. Unfortunately, if this insincere behaviour is accepted by others, it will be expected to be repeated in similar circumstances. If others realise that the person is being insincere, then the very rejection they feared in the first place can actually occur.

One of the cornerstones of building a rapport with others is by being honest or genuine with them (Rogers 1980). This genuineness means there will be times when an individual disagrees with others, but it helps to develop a more positive approach knowing that by being honest with others one is being honest with oneself.

A nurse who displays incongruity towards a patient through a mismatch of verbal and non-verbal signals or by saying something that seems false, will, according to Smith (1992), cause the patient to become confused and suspicious. Above all, the patient will question the credibility of the nurse and may find it difficult to maintain a relationship. A nurse who is genuine is likely to be perceived by the patient as trustworthy and capable of receiving a confidence.

Activity 4.2 Genuine and incongruent behaviour

Observe the interactions of others during the next week. Note when a person is being genuine. What verbal and non-verbal behaviour leads you to this conclusion ?

Similarly, using the same criteria, note when a person is being incongruent.

So far this chapter has examined typical interactions and pointed out some of the factors that might lead to misunderstanding and misinterpretation. Much of this is due to the beliefs, values, attitudes, prejudices and so on of the parties involved in the interaction. The next part of the chapter will deal with these aspects in more detail.

COMMUNICATION FILTERS

Communication filters are often referred to in earlier texts as barriers. However, this word would seem to indicate that they create a complete block to incoming information. In reality, the information is distorted or filtered rather than blocked. There are many possible factors that may act as filters to communication and the ones that commonly occur are listed in Box 4.2 and are described in more detail below.

DEFENCE MECHANISMS

When a person behaves in an unexpected way, usually displaying extreme emotions such as anger or sorrow, it is said that 'his defences are down' or 'he is showing his true colours'. The 'defences' referred to are unconscious motivations described by Anna Freud (1946), the daughter of Sigmund Freud. Everyday phrases such as 'having repressed feelings' or 'having a fixation' about something are taken from psychoanalytical terminology.

According to Freud's theory an individual's personality is made up of three parts:

* The id
* The ego
* The superego

The id represents the unconscious, instinctual desires that are unrestrained—self gratification is the goal. However, when interacting with others, it is not always socially acceptable to satisfy one's desires. A restraining force needs to operate and this is the role of the 'ego'. The 'ego' modifies the instinctual urges of the 'id' so that the person is able to interact in a socially acceptable way.

However, within these structures there is still no moral code, no guilt or shame. The third structure that achieves this is known as the 'superego' or conscience.

The development of these three components of the personality can be seen in a child from infancy to about 4 years of age, according to Sigmund Freud (1954). The infant reacts with basic instinctual drives and is completely self-centred. At around 2-3 years of age, the child begins to relate to others and modifies his desires according to the reinforcements he obtains from the parent, such as chastisement or praise.

As the child develops language, phrases such as 'Don't do that', 'Do as you are told' and 'It's naughty to hit your brother' impart a set of preferred behaviours to him. This learning and internalising of preferred behaviours is termed socialisation and can continue to develop and be modified throughout life.

As long as the person's well-being is intact, the ego and superego will work together to modify or hold in check the basic instinctual urges of the id. However, when a person's well-being is under threat, to avoid the id breaking through and causing irresponsible behaviour, or the superego breaking through leading to overwhelming feelings of guilt, the ego enlists defence mechanisms to counteract this.

Nearly 20 defence mechanisms have been described, but they all have the same characteristics according to Emslie (1979). These are that:

* Self-esteem is maintained.
* Anxiety and guilt are reduced.
* There is an indirect liberation of instinctual expression in an unconscious way.

Some of the more common defence mechanisms that have been described are listed in Box 4.3 and are described briefly below.

Box 4.2 Communication filters

* Defence mechanisms
* Attitudes, beliefs and values
* Attributions and assumptions
* Prejudices
* Perceptual distortions

Box 4.3 Common defence mechanisms

* Rationalisation
* Regression
* Repression
* Denial
* Identification
* Projection
* Fantasy

Rationalisation

Rationalisation occurs when an individual gives reasons for behaviour that, to the individual, seem perfectly reasonable. For example, a student states that he will start work on his essay as soon as he has watched the 'important' documentary on television.

Phrases such as 'I'll give up smoking as soon as I pass the exam' or the man who says 'the relationship was heading for the rocks anyway' as his girlfriend leaves are other examples where the person wants something to occur but can't achieve it.

The nurse, who having repeatedly ignored the patient's call buzzer because she doesn't like to talk to him, states 'I'm so busy with the care plans that I can't see to him now'.

Regression

Regression is characterised by behaviour appropriate to an earlier stage of development. Thumb sucking by an adult is a mild form of this. Bedwetting by an older child after a change in a familiar environment, such as going into hospital, is another example.

An extreme example occurs in some forms of mental illness such as depression when a patient may curl up in a corner in the foetal position, regressing back to the womb.

Repression

Repression is an unconscious submerging of memories and feelings by an individual, usually of past events, to avoid anxiety or guilt feelings.

The person who witnesses the results of a terrorist bomb attack, or is involved in an armed conflict may lose partial or total memory of the events. However, the memories are still there and can lead to physical symptoms such as tiredness and weakness.

Denial

Denial is an unconscious defence mechanism used by an individual against anxiety inducing events, even in the face of such events. For example, loss of consciousness or fainting when receiving an emotional shock is a form of denial. Denial is seen most frequently when there is grief or severe loss either of a person, or a body part such as amputation of a limb. The widow who sets the table at home for two and states 'Frank will be home soon from work. He always likes his tea on the table' is exhibiting a severe form of denial.

Identification

Identification is admiration of another person to the point of taking on some of the characteristics of that person. Usually, the person is famous and may be a film star, a sportsperson or a well known public figure. Some theorists believe that by identifying with a particular character on film, a sort of catharsis, or release of primitive instinctual urges takes place in a safe, controlled way.

Others dispute this however, by stating that the more a person is exposed to violence and sex on film or TV the more likely they are to take on these behaviours themselves. For a review of the research into this area see Glover (1985).

Projection

Projection occurs when a person's undesirable traits are attributed to, or projected upon, others to avoid punishment. Thus the person who has an unconscious prejudice against someone of another race, may project those feelings onto a second person, accusing them of being a bigot.

Fantasy

Fantasy is the use of the imagination to conjure up an image of something that is desired by an individual. Usually, the object or person is unobtainable. Most people engage in fantasy. It can be used as a means of stress reduction, such as imagining being on a beach in the sun with the rhythmic sound of the waves breaking on the shore. However, too much time spent in fantasy means that less time is spent in reality. This can lead to daydreaming and non-attentive behaviour, and is obviously undesirable where others are involved.

Defence mechanisms may have a short-term beneficial effect in maintaining self-esteem and reducing anxiety and guilt. However, if overused, they can cause severe distortions of reality in that they can affect the way an individual perceives and interacts with others.

ATTITUDES, BELIEFS AND VALUES

A person's beliefs and values strongly predict what attitude will be adopted to a particular event. An individual's attitude is observable by others in the form of behaviour, whereas beliefs and values are not.

According to Adler & Rodman (1991):

1. An attitude is a response to something in either a positive or a negative way.
2. A belief is a conviction of the right of something based on cultural upbringing.
3. A value is at the core of the person. It is a belief in the worth of a concept. Values are usually embodied in complex moral or religious systems that are found in all cultures and societies.

Activity 4.3   Attitudes, beliefs and values

In this activity think of your attitudes towards college, work, politics and sport. Make a statement about each area down one side of the page and on the other side list the people or groups that have influenced your attitude and the way in which they did this. Which attitudes were more difficult to describe in terms of their origin and why ?

Attitudes, beliefs and values are acquired: a person is not born with them. Most fundamental beliefs and values are gained from those who influence the individual most—parents, siblings, teachers, friends and media figures.

Children are rewarded for displaying the 'right' attitude and punished for displaying the 'wrong' one. Eventually, through positive or negative reinforcement (see Ch. 2) the behaviour will either continue, or become extinguished.

Children also take on the behaviour or attitudes of role models by observation and imitation. Parents are amongst the most important role models, but television personalities or cartoon characters can also have a strong effect. Media use has been made of Superman to impress upon children that the habit of smoking is bad for health.

According to Niven (1989), research on attitude formation shows that attitudes towards health are best influenced in the formative years and are more lasting. Therefore health education should start at an early age. Parents and the media are in an ideal position to achieve this.

It is through socialisation and interpersonal communication that people develop attitudes, beliefs and values. These in turn effect the unique way in which a person views the world. It is this uniqueness that acts as a filter to communication and can lead to misunderstanding and misinterpretation. People who have the same basic concept of something don't always believe in it the same way. For example, two people may express a belief that waste should be recycled, yet only one takes used paper and bottles to the waste banks.

Someone may hold a belief that smoking is a bad habit and yet continue to smoke. This can generate frustration and anger among health care staff when the patient is readmitted for a third time during winter suffering with chronic bronchitis.

Changing people's attitudes

Health professionals are involved daily in attempting to change people's attitudes. Knowledge of how attitudes are changed would therefore be useful. According to Kagan et al (1986) it is the need in most people to maintain consistency, that is the key to attitude change. Theorists state that attitudes have three components:

- A thinking component (cognitive).
- An emotional component (affective).
- An action component (conative).

Change occurring in any one of these three should bring about a change in the others. See the example in Box 4.4.

If the patient described in Box 4.4 is advised by health care staff, or other patients, that smoking has a definite effect on heart disease, it will create

---

Box 4.4 The three components of attitude

A man with heart disease may continue to smoke, despite advice from all sources to give up. If this patient considered that smoking was hazardous, his attitude could be characterised by thoughts, feelings and actions that are consistent with each other. 'I think (cognition) that smoking is insignificant as a cause of my heart condition. I like smoking (affective). I will carry on smoking (conative)'.

---

inconsistency or tension within the system and there will be an attempt to reduce the habit. This state of tension is known as cognitive dissonance (Festinger 1957). When faced with this dilemma, several courses of action could take place.

The man could change his attitude towards smoking so that it is consistent with this new information. He could seek out new information that is consistent with his current attitude, such as reports of studies suggesting smoking has few or no ill effects. Or he could cite a relative who lived to 90 years of age and smoked all his life.

Lastly, the smoker could minimise or reduce the importance of the inconsistency by ignoring the leaflets or advice. 'It's the only pleasure I have in life. We all have to die from something'. Nurses therefore, may need to be particularly persuasive in their attempts to change attitudes.

Persuasive messages

According to Niven (1989) there are three elements of persuasive messages:

- The characteristics of the communicator.
- The communication itself.
- The characteristics of the recipient.

The communicator

The communicator must be credible and a recognised expert. A first year student nurse who states that regular exercise is important for physical well-being would have less impact than a consultant physician or a top sports personality.

The communication

The message may be emotional or fear inducing in which case the appeal should be strong.

Individuals must believe that they are at risk if they ignore the message and that the danger will pass if they follow the advice.

The message may appeal to reason, whereby a one or two-sided argument can be put forward. In the example of the smoker, a two-sided argument would probably work better, presenting the evidence from both perspectives and highlighting the flaws in the pro-smoking argument.

Use of appropriate humour is essential in making a message stick in the mind of a patient or client. This is evident in the field of advertising where annual awards are given to those judged the most humorous.

Methods of presenting information will influence groups or individuals in different ways. Some people will respond readily to visual communication of film or demonstration whilst others may prefer the written or spoken word.

The recipient

Kagan et al (1986) and Niven (1989) have discussed the characteristics of the recipient of the message. It was thought that people with a low self-esteem were more likely to be persuaded than those with a high self-esteem. However, more recently, cognitive arguments have been put forward. These claim that a person is less likely to change his mind if he is able to think of a number of counter-arguments to the message. Sometimes a person will go out of his way to do the opposite of what he has been told so as not to appear to have lost the right to think for himself.

For the health professional to deliver a persuasive message, it is necessary to have an awareness of how a person's attitudes, beliefs and values will influence the reception of that message. The professional's value system is not necessarily the same as that of the patient.

ATTRIBUTIONS AND ASSUMPTIONS

People often make assumptions about each other on very flimsy evidence, such as the type of clothing worn, style of speaking, and the role held in society.

A certain amount of labelling occurs as a result of such assumptions. For example, a man wearing a clerical collar will be labelled as religious, pious, a paragon of virtue, a comforter and counsellor. If these labels are reinforced enough by others, then the individual may begin to take on these characteristics in excess. This is known as a self-fulfilling prophecy.

Activity 4.4 Attributions and assumptions

List any changes in your behaviour since you became a student nurse on one side of a piece of paper. On the other side, explain why these changes have occured. What does this say about labelling and the self-fulfilling prophecy ?

Labelling can lead to stereotyping whereby people are slotted into neat pigeon-holes. This mechanism helps maintain consistency and when something occurs to change the label or stereotype, cognitive dissonance occurs.

The clergyman who is reported in the press as having an affair with one of his parishioners will immediately undergo a label change. The blame will be laid fully on him by an outraged public because he betrayed the stereotype of a typical clergyman.

The fault will lie with him rather than with some other external agency (i.e. the woman, his wife, or the pressures of his job). Fritz Heider (1958) has suggested that when observing behaviour, individuals attempt to use a cause and effect analysis to make sense of it. He has described two types of cause:

- Dispositional (personal).
- Situational (environmental).

People tend to attribute dispositional causes to others when something goes wrong, and attribute situational causes to themselves. When one person sees another fall down the stairs, clumsiness may be seen as the cause. If, however, the same thing happens to the observer, a loose carpet may be blamed.

When attempting to account for behaviour, an individual is more apt to attribute negative behaviours to environmental factors and positive behaviours to personal factors. For example 'I was angry because the carpet was loose' or,'he was so clumsy, I had to go and help him up'.

The problem with such assumptions is that in the case of the other person falling over, the situational factors such as a loose carpet, slippery shoes, or an object on the stairs is not taken into account; the context of the behaviour is ignored. This is known as attribution error. An area where attribution theory is reversed is in the case of clinical depression.

Rather than attribute negative behaviour to situational factors, the depressed person will blame himself. Positive behaviour is attributed to situational factors, often temporary, yet very specific, such as, 'I ate my breakfast today because it was a cereal I like.'

PREJUDICES

Prejudice involves making assumptions about people and attributing certain labels and stereotypes to them. Prejudice can be seen in many aspects of life, often in relation to:

- Race
- Colour
- Religion
- Politics
- Sexual orientation
- Marital status
- Hair colour
- Type or style of clothing
- Height
- Weight
- Age

Many job application forms now have two sections, one for career information, the other for personal information. The two sections are separated before going to the shortlisting panel so that a decision is based solely on the career section. Despite this, prejudices still surface.

One panel member may dislike writing that slopes to the left and therefore discriminate against that candidate, probably in an unconscious way.

Prejudices are often related to stereotypes and involve what appear to others to be illogical and emotional thoughts and actions but which are quite logical to the individual concerned. The object of the prejudice is different in some way from the 'norm', as perceived by the individual who labels the object. For example, a white Englishman could be non prejudiced against a white Dutchman yet be prejudiced against another Englishman who happens to be black.

Hardy & Heyes (1987) have described an experiment carried out in a primary school by the teacher, Jane Elliot (see Box 4.5).

What the experiments described in Box 4.5 demonstrate is how irrational and discriminatory prejudices are. Much of the research into how prejudices can be reduced has shown that if intergroup teams are constructed, with equal status in the group between members, and common goals to work towards, then reductions do occur.

To achieve a reduction in prejudice in the nursing environment is potentially difficult because of the mix of grades. However, if each person in the team is made to feel that they have an equal contribution to make to the running of the ward or unit, then prejudices will be reduced.

Box 4.5   Prejudice

A teacher, Jane Elliot, told her class of 9-year-olds that those with brown eyes were more intelligent than those with blue eyes (she had blue eyes herself). Rules were laid down, such as the 'inferior' students were to sit at the back of the class and use proper cups instead of the drinking fountain. The 'superior' students were given extra privileges. The blue-eyed children although in the majority, became depressed, angry and sullen. They attributed negative words to themselves such as dull and stupid. This became a self-fulfilling prophecy in a remarkably short time (within minutes). The blue-eyed children became nasty and vicious.

The next day, Mrs Elliot stated she had made a mistake, and that it was really the brown-eyed children who were inferior. Almost immediately they reverted to the same behaviour as the blue-eyed children the day before. An interesting point was that many of the brown-eyed children also had black skin, but this was disregarded by the white children in the fight against the common enemy.

This same experiment has been repeated in a more sophisticated form with adults, with similar results. The experiment raised a number of ethical questions and for this reason, participants were fully debriefed on each occasion, resulting in a mixture of relief and laughter.

To be more successful, this concept would need to involve all members of the multidisciplinary team, including the patient.

In this situation individual prejudices can be submerged in striving for the common goal. However, they could still surface unconsciously in the ways in which a nurse might interact non-verbally with a patient. For example, the patient may be referred to as:

• The child-batterer.
• The patient with scar tissue of face or hands.
• The patient with a different religious viewpoint.
• The demanding patient.

It is useful to reflect on prejudices and to devise strategies to reduce them.

PERCEPTUAL DISTORTIONS

In order to pay attention, the perception of a stimulus needs to occur, and yet distortions can happen. Perception is extremely selective. If it were not, there would be a hopeless jumble of sounds, scents, sights and sensations, all competing for attention and causing sensory overload.

Activity 4.5   Perceptual distortions

Sit in a chair in a familiar room. Have someone else sit in another chair. Both close your eyes for two minutes. Concentrate on the sounds within and around you, in the room and outside. When you open your eyes, write down all the things you heard and compare your list with the other person. You will notice many similarities but also some differences.

In Activity 4.5 although two people might hear the same sounds, each will be selective in their perception of that sound. The chances are that a sound which is heard outside the room illicits the response 'It sounds like. . . . '.

The brain has to rely on incoming information via the senses to identify what is a stimulus. It is constantly comparing a sound, smell, sight or touch with the 'memory bank' of similar sensations.

If a loud bang is heard outside, the response could be 'that sounds like a car backfiring'. Another person hearing the same sound may say 'that sounds like a gun being fired'. Each person hears the same sound, yet 'perceives' it differently. Without being present to see what caused the sound, each individual makes an assumption based on his past experience of the same or a similar sound and each individual defines what the sound is almost before it is 'heard'.

Activity 4.6   Anticipating stimuli

The anticipation of a stimuli is called a perceptual set. In the following sentence count how many times the letter F appears.

Forty four people were of more than average build in the scientific study carried out of teenage school children.

In Activity 4.6, most people identify three 'F's. Actually there are five. The 'F' in 'of' sounds like a 'v' and so disappears. Perception of the outside world is similar enough for most people to enable them to communicate using common definitions (e.g. red, tree, B. flat). However, it is wrong to assume that what one person 'sees' is always what everyone else 'sees'. The magician's illusion is a classical example.

The audience 'see' the assistant disappearing from the box, but another magician will see a false panel knowing how the trick is done. The audience know that the assistant hasn't really disappeared because they have seen the trick performed before. However, the illusion is so strong, that it still causes the brain to perceive an impossible event. The second magician, because of his training, was able to perceive things that the audience did not. Similarly, an experienced nurse, a student nurse and a patient will perceive the same stimuli in different ways, based on their level of understanding, beliefs, values and past experiences. All the factors mentioned in this chapter can contribute to differing interpretations of the same event.

A patient who is having a surgical wound redressed for the first time, may perceive all the equipment as threatening and may anticipate a considerable amount of pain. A student nurse would perceive this situation as an opportunity to practise her newly acquired skills of aseptic technique, and would be concentrating on remembering the sequence of cleansing the wound and manipulating the forceps. An experienced nurse would perceive the situation as an opportunity to converse with the patient, to put him at ease and assess the condition of the wound. The nurse would then determine what action to take in relation to the dressing of the wound, based on her experience of other similar wounds. Each of the three persons have different perceptual sets of the same stimuli.

All these factors show ways in which an individual filters incoming stimuli from the world and creates a unique view of that world. People do interact with each other in different contexts and it is the effects of these contexts, which are now discussed.

COMMUNICATION IN CONTEXT

In the previous section, the way in which an individual perceives certain stimuli was discussed. This perception is influenced by the context. For example the symbol 13 can be perceived as the letter B or the number 13 depending upon the context (A B C D or 12 13 14 15).

Describing the context in which communication takes place uses an interactionist approach. It takes into account not only internal factors, but also the role perceptions of the people involved and the external constraints imposed upon the interaction. Baron & Byrne (1991) cite the example of a woman who becomes pregnant. The woman may see this as an 'accident'. The obstetrician who runs a fertility clinic may, on the other hand, see this as successful high fertility on the part of the woman and her husband. The same behaviour is attributed to different causes, depending on who is observing it.

Alternatively, behaviour could be modified according to the context. An office worker would probably communicate differently at a formal dinner party with his boss, than when eating a pub lunch with a group of friends.

Another aspect of context is the way in which people remember certain events. Memories of events are not a random set of mental associations, but a recreation of the context of that event. This is known by cognitive psychologists as context-dependent coding, and is best illustrated through hearing a favourite tune.

Memories of where the tune was first heard, what the person was doing, and even emotions associated with it come flooding back.

CULTURE IN CONTEXT

People from differing cultures are coming together more and more as world travel becomes increasingly accessible. It is important therefore to consider the way in which culture influences communication.

In the last 30 years, much research has been carried out into the way in which culture affects communication, particularly in non-verbal communication. For a more comprehensive discussion of this area see Argyle (1988) and Morris (1976).

The complexities of non-verbal communication in different cultures create a potential mine field with respect to common understanding. For example, if a left-handed British person were to hold out his left hand to shake hands when meeting a Moslem, he would greatly insult the Moslem because, in the latter's culture, this is the hand that is used for, and is therefore associated with, cleaning up after excretion.

Public bodily contact between acquaintances, for example embracing and kissing, is not the norm in Britain whereas it is common in French and Latin cultures. Arabs and Latin Americans stand in close proximity to one another when conversing, yet Swedes and Scots are more distant. The gesture for 'O.K.' in Britain is usually a circle formed by the thumb and index finger, with the other fingers pointing upwards. To a Tunisian this same signal means 'I am going to kill you'. In some cultures respect for another is shown by avoiding direct eye contact, whereas in other cultures, this lack of eye contact would indicate lack of interest, or suggest that the individual was being dishonest.

The use of silence in communication varies between cultures and sometimes within cultures.

In the western world, silence in conversation is viewed in a negative way. It tends to indicate unwillingness to communicate or lack of interest. In eastern cultures however, silence is frequently used and the expression of thoughts and feelings is discouraged. This can create problems when people from an eastern culture apply for jobs with a western company. When asked at interview to discuss thoughts or feelings, or to express themselves, they would have great difficulty. To do so readily would be a sign of insincerity or boasting. Lack of eye contact might lead the interviewer to perceive that they were under-confident.

Emotional expression varies between cultures. For example, a British person who receives a telephone call to say his mother has died may stand up and excuse himself from the meeting he has been attending. An Italian would probably be more demonstrative in the expression of his sudden grief.

Funerals are characterised by differences in expression of emotion. The British reaction to any pain, either physical or emotional, is to remain calm and to keep the emotions under control. However, the Latin approach is to express emotions freely. In some Asian cultures there are women whose function both before and after funerals, is to wail loudly over the body of the deceased. This is both accepted and expected behaviour.

These examples may be over-generalisations and it is important that nurses should avoid falling into the trap of stereotyping and labelling people from different cultures.

This perception can be generalised to any patient who doesn't fit into the role of the ideal patient, a person who is quiet, cooperative and undemanding. The effect of the non-stereotypical patient is documented in research carried out by Stockwell (1972). She found that patients were likely to be avoided by nurses if they were non-British, in hospital for more than 3 months, or who regularly questioned their care and did not comply with routines.

Such unpopular patients did not receive individual holistic care. They were labelled nuisances or hypochondriacs. This could even lead to the withholding of medication to control pain. The more popular, uncomplaining patient could receive better pain control than the very expressive patient. When a behaviour is seen in context, misinterpretation about why the behaviour is taking place can be avoided.

IMPLICATIONS FOR PRACTICE

Communication is a complex process involving both interpersonal and intrapersonal factors. Each person is a unique individual, with a unique interpretation of the world, influenced by origin, upbringing and life experience.

Is an individual's personality shaped by genetic, hereditary factors (nature), or is it shaped by the environment in which he lives (nurture)? Most Schools of Psychology offer arguments in favour of one approach or the other although some may believe both to be important (see Box 4.6).

What seems certain is the lack of simple conclusive answers to describe the uniqueness of the individual, although some factors, particularly internal ones, can be described. For example:

- Defence mechanisms
- Attitudes
- Assumptions
- Prejudices
- Perceptual distortions

These factors modify external stimuli and determine the way in which a person will respond to them. The physical and cultural contexts of the interaction are also important.

Nurses need to be aware of these factors and be able to see them in themselves as well as in their patients/clients. This will help them to empathise and interact in a meaningful way with others. The concept of self-awareness and the skills involved in successful communication will be discussed in Chapter 5.

In the following example taken from an authentic situation it is possible to identify some of the areas that have been discussed in this chapter. The skill is to determine ways in which the outcome described here could have been avoided.

Box 4.6   Nature or nurture?

1. The biological approach favours nature and believes it to comprise biological systems which are only partially influenced by the environment.
2. The behaviourist approach stresses the effect of the environment and persons within it as the source of reward and punishment. It is therefore on the side of nurture.
3. The cognitive approach suggests that the debate about nature and nurture is irrelevant. Both have equal input into the way an individual perceives the world.
4. The humanist approach of Rogers and Maslow emphasises that nature and nurture are merely boundaries within which human nature is free to develop to its full potential.
5. The psychodynamic approach reinforces the impact of the effects of the environment upon the unconscious behaviour of the person.

Box 4.7   Miscommunication

Staff Nurse Murphy was arriving on the night shift in the operating theatre. She was told by the departing staff nurse that the theatre needed preparing for Dr. Ahmed, who was operating on Abraham Liddle first thing in the morning. When the staff nurse left, Nurse Murphy realised that she had not been told what operation the patient was having. She rang round the wards to find out about Abraham Liddle. All the wards she contacted had no patient by that name. By now the time was 12 midnight. Staff Nurse Murphy decided to call the surgeon. Dr. Ahmed had been asleep for 1 hour when the telephone rang.

He was upset at being woken over such a trivial matter, and at such a late hour, when he needed sleep. He answered the nurse sharply, stating that of course the patient existed, he had examined him that afternoon and he did not want to be disturbed again. He then banged the 'phone down. The Staff Nurse, upset and angry at the doctor's response to a perfectly reasonable request, attempted to locate the patient again, without success. She prepared the theatre for general surgery as best she could.

The next night she returned to duty to be confronted by an irate theatre sister, who stated that the theatre list had been held up for an hour that morning, because the Abraham Needle which Dr. Ahmed had needed to carry out a liver biopsy on his first patient, Mr. Johnstone, was not available as had been requested.

CONCLUSION

Communication is about being aware of the way in which messages can be influenced by all the factors discussed. A way of checking one's own perception is by the use of metacommunication and feedback. By doing this, other people in the interaction will perceive that they are relating to someone, who, as Carl Rogers would say, is showing unconditional positive regard and empathetic understanding.

REFERENCES

Adler R B, Rodman G 1991 Understanding human communication, 4th edn. Holt, Rinehart, Winston, Florida.

Argyle M 1988 Bodily communication, 2nd edn. Methuen, London.

Baron R A, Byrne D 1991 Social psychology—understanding human interactions, 6th edn. Simon, Schuster, Needham Heights, U.S.A.

Emslie G R 1979 The psychoanalytical approach. In: Medcof J, Roth J (eds) Approaches to psychology. Open University Press, Milton Keynes.

Festinger L 1957 A theory of cognitive dissonance. Paterson, Evanston Row.

Freud A 1946 The ego and mechanisms of defence. International Universities Press.

Freud S 1954 The origins of psychoanalysis. Basic Books, New York.

Glover D 1985 The sociology of the mass media. In: Haralambos M (ed) Sociology new directions. Causeway Press, Ormskirk.

Hagie O (ed) 1986 A handbook of communication skills. Routledge, London.

Hardy M, Heyes S 1987 Beginning psychology, 3rd edn. Weidenfield, Nicholson, London.

Heider F 1958 The psychology of interpersonal relations. Wiley, New York.

Kagan C, Evans J & Kay B 1986 A manual of interpersonal skills for nurses—an experiential approach. Harper & Row, London.

Maslow A 1954 Motivation and personality. Harper & Row, New York.

Morris D 1975 Manwatching. Cape, London.

Niven N 1989 Health psychology. Churchill Livingstone, Edinburgh.

Oxford English Dictionary 1988 University Press, Oxford.

Pluckman M L 1978 Human communication: the matrix of nursing. McGraw Hill, New York.

Rogers C R 1961 On becoming a person. Houghton Mifflin, Boston.

Rogers C R 1980 A way of being. Houghton Mifflin, Boston.

Smith S 1992 Communications in nursing, 2nd edn. Mosby, St Louis.

Stockwell F 1972 The unpopular patient. Royal College of Nursing, London.

Waalen J K 1979 A comparison of approaches. In: Medcof J, Roth J (eds) Approaches to psychology. Open University Press, Milton Keynes.

5

Improving communication

Andy Betts

INTRODUCTION

When two people engage in conversation much more is taking place than the observer sees. Each person brings his own unique world and perceptions to the encounter in which a multi-faceted and apparently infinite collection of stimuli and data are involved. It is hard to imagine how people could proceed through everyday life if they were to pay attention to every minute detail of communication. The human brain instantaneously and efficiently filters the thousands of cues and messages thus preventing the overloading of data. This filtering process is not predominantly a conscious activity. In this chapter we identify those factors that cause problems in communication and we focus on what may be done to improve the effectiveness of communication in nursing.

COMMUNICATION AND HEALTH CARE

Studies over the last two decades identify communication problems as persistent causes for concern in the delivery of health care (Menzies 1970, Stockwell 1972, Hayward 1975, Macleod-Clark 1984, Faulkner 1985, Ley 1988). Nursing curricula have been modified in response to these findings but there remains little room for complacency.

The reasons for the problems are complex and often specific to the area being researched. Those commonly cited include: lack of skills and training, lack of resources and time, emotional vulnerability, the location of power, and some deliberately perpetuated bad practices between agencies. Perhaps this is no different to the picture in other fields of human encounter when one considers the complexities of communication. Also, the context in which nursing takes place is an elaborate network of relationships with patients, colleagues, informal carers and allied agencies. The potential for things to go wrong is great.

Peplau (1988) suggests that nursing is essentially an interpersonal process. If this is the case, then competent nurses are required to be effective communicators and each nurse has a responsibility to pay adequate attention to his own development in this domain. This chapter is grounded in the belief that individuals can become more effective communicators. The pursuit of perfection in communication is a frustrating process. Frustrating because it is lifelong and everyday experiences serve to remind us just how complex and elusive effective communication actually is. Frustrating because to become more effective requires a realisation of inadequacies.

THE NATURE OF THE PROBLEM

There are four major factors that contribute to communication problems in nursing:

- Lack of self-awareness.
- Lack of systematic interpersonal skills training.
- Lack of a conceptual framework.
- Lack of clarity of purpose.

These factors will each be examined in turn.

Lack of self-awareness

One reason why communication may be ineffective is the lack of awareness of aspects of oneself which significantly affect interactions with others. Facets of the individual which are beyond consciousness are also beyond control and become 'loose cannons' which may blow a hole in the best of intentions. The personal factors which affect communication are attitudes, values,

---

Box 5.1 Increasing self-awareness

Julie, a student on the learning disabilities branch, watches the replay of a video recording of herself interacting with a fellow student. She is both fascinated and disconcerted by what she observes. Seeing herself from the outside presents a contrasting image to the 'internal' view she has of herself.

She notices repeated mannerisms which previously she had no idea she used. She is able to check out later with her peers how they had experienced these behaviours and is not too surprised to discover that they had been perceived as a distraction by others. As a result of this experience Julie is aware of aspects of herself which were previously beyond her consciousness. This learning experience has increased her options and further refined her capacity to communicate effectively with others.

---

beliefs, feelings and behaviours. Increasing self-awareness in these domains is likely to result in more productive interactions and a more intentional use of self. This increased self understanding serves to convert potential pitfalls into potential assets.

The realisation that the image one has of oneself may contrast significantly with how one is perceived by others is significant learning and lies at the heart of developing as a communicator. Individuals tend to acquire a subjective view of the world which is different to how others perceive it and much of behaviour is partly unconsciously motivated. Both of these observations mean that nurses, who are directly involved in interpersonal relationships, need to maximise their self-awareness and conscious use of self. Stein-Parbury (1993) states:

Nurses need to develop acute self-awareness whenever they engage in interactions and relationships with patients, because the primary tool they are using in these circumstances is themselves. Without self-awareness nurses run the risk of imposing their values and views onto patients…Through self-awareness nurses remain in touch with what they are doing and how this is affecting patients for whom they care.

(Stein-Parbury, p.60)

One important characteristic of human communication is that not all signals and messages are sent intentionally or even consciously (see Chapter 1). There is often a discrepancy between what the individual perceives during communication and other people's understanding. This has important implications for the nurse as a communicator because it is this potential discrepancy which leads to all kinds of problems in communication. Effective communication requires people to maximise self-awareness, both in terms of how behaviour is perceived by others and also in understanding one's own motivations and blind spots.

Lack of systematic interpersonal skills training

The use of the words 'systematic' and 'training' is highly significant and controversial in the context of interpersonal skills. To some degree communication consists of a set of skills. These are the 'tools of the trade of communication'. As such, the most effective method of becoming competent in using them is the same as for any skills training. Of course, communication is much more than a technology but systematic skills training has a role to play in becoming an effective communicator. There is a reluctance to accept this notion for fear that communication will, in some way, be reduced to a dehumanised series of mechanistic behaviours and formulae. This does not apply to other aspects of the nurse's role such as carrying out complex clinical procedures. In these cases the skills are practised until competence is achieved.

Systematic interpersonal skills training, if structured correctly, does not result in homogenised cloning but competent communicators who have integrated identified skills into their unique style of communication. The systematic training in the use of microskills is just the first step in a process that must lead to these skills becoming second nature (Patterson 1988).

Chapter 1 includes some description of human development and a clue as to why things may go wrong is revealed by the question 'how do people learn to communicate?' An important part of a child's development is to learn to communicate effectively. How does this happen in practice? Surprisingly, it is left largely to chance. It is acquired mainly from parents, the significant role models in early life, and also from other influential grown ups and peers. It would appear that this learning process works amazingly well. The capabilities of even a pre-school child to communicate using a wide ranging vocabulary are impressive. By the age of physical maturity most are capable of a complex repertoire of interactions.

On a different level, however, it is possible to be critical of the absence of systematic interpersonal skills training. If, as seems to be the case, children acquire skills as they go along it would appear that they are also likely to learn some of the 'bad habits' of their role models and lack the awareness necessary to discriminate between what is effective and what is not. The consequences for nursing are significant. Egan (1990) notes that those entering the helping professions often do not possess the basic set of helping skills. Historically, nursing curricula have failed to address this deficit although there has been an increasing emphasis on interpersonal skills training in recent years with varying degrees of success (Dunn 1991).

Lack of a conceptual framework

Nurses who demonstrate competence in the application of interpersonal skills may sometimes use them in an ad hoc fashion (Dunn 1991). A theoretical framework is required which informs communication and provides a structure for the analysis, reflection and evaluation of interactions. Given the complexities highlighted in previous chapters, attempting to understand communication without a framework is problematic. It is important for nurses to be able to conceptualise what they are doing to ensure that skills are used in a coherent and strategic manner. Such a framework provides the language and organisation to make sense of interactions both retrospectively and as they occur. Although many different theories and models exist to explain different aspects of the nurse's role e.g. nursing care models, counselling models, management models and supervision models, there are far fewer theories designed to focus solely on communication. Two such theories will be considered later in this chapter.

Lack of clarity of purpose

On a conscious level communication is concerned with making choices. The effective communicator has a high success rate of making appropriate choices for the situations that are encountered because he is clear about the aims or purpose of each interaction (Heron 1990). This enables the effective communicator to discriminate between alternative choices, selecting what suits a specific situation. It is not usually the nurse who determines the purpose of the interaction but the needs of the client. This process requires sensitivity and empathy (see Chapter 9) to enable the nurse to read the situation accurately and assess what is required. For example, the communication skills required in giving advice on a specific subject are significantly different to those required to listen to a distressed individual. Developing the ability to read situations, to be clear about the intention and to pursue it strategically are the hallmarks of effective communication.

IMPROVING COMMUNICATION BY ADDRESSING DEFICITS

INCREASING SELF-AWARENESS

Burnard (1985) defines self-awareness as a process. He says:

Self-awareness refers to the gradual and continuous process of noticing and exploring aspects of self, whether behavioural, psychological or physical, with the intention of developing personal and interpersonal understanding... to have a deeper understanding of ourselves is to have a sharper and clearer picture of what is happening to others. In a sense it is a process of discrimination.

(Burnard, 1985, pp. 15-16)

This concept of discrimination is linked to ideas discussed in Chapter 1, in the context of internal and external worlds. Recognising differences and similarities to others is an important aspect of work in human care services.

Rogers (1967) emphasised that understanding oneself is a significant pre-requisite to understanding others. How is this achieved? Indeed, is

it achievable? The idea that self-awareness can be achieved on a certain day may sound ridiculous. The concept of self-awareness is best thought of as a continuum. The lifelong task is to inch along that continuum in the realisation and acceptance that the end may never be reached. Any progress made is through introspective processes such as reflection, self exploration and self assessment and by interactive activities such as self disclosure, discussion and feedback. In addition, some may choose to enter a counselling or psychotherapeutic relationship in a deliberate attempt to heighten self-awareness (see Chapter 9).

Learning through reflection

The term 'reflective practitioner' now appears frequently within nursing literature (Schon 1983). Nurses seek to incorporate reflection into their practice but confusion exists regarding the meaning of the word. Boud et al (1985) state quite succinctly that reflection in this context refers to 'turning experience into learning'. This is a purposeful and conscious activity requiring structured time and effort rather than an automatic process. Different methods can be used to achieve this, such as introspection, writing or discussion. One common misconception of reflection is that it consists purely of historical analysis (see Fig. 5.1). Kemmis (1985) stresses that reflection is not an end in itself but that it leads to informed, committed action. Development as a reflective communicator eventually leads to the ability to process what is happening during an interaction rather than after it has finished. Accurate processing of communication as it occurs increases options and results in a more intentional use of self.

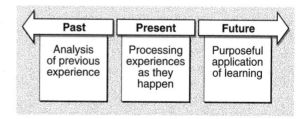

Figure 5.1 Three dimensions of reflection

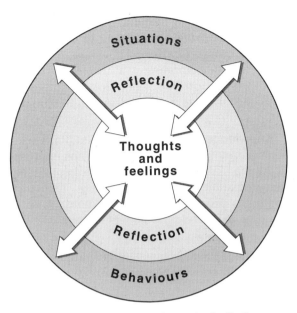

Situations

Reflection

Thoughts and feelings

Reflection

Behaviours

Figure 5.2 Internal and external aspects of reflection

Box 5.2 Examples of reflective questions

What was the context of the interaction?
What actually happened?
What was my reaction to what happened?
What were my behaviours, thoughts, feelings at the time?
What was the behaviour of the other(s)?
What do I imagine were the other'(s) thoughts and feelings at the time?
What were my thoughts and feelings afterwards?
What do I imagine were the other'(s) thoughts and feelings afterwards?
What was the purpose of the interaction?
How successful was the interaction?
What skills did I use well/not so well?
Given the opportunity how would I do it differently?

Reflection involves both inward and outward activities (see Fig. 5.2). The inward activity is concerned with paying attention to thoughts and feelings and the external focus is on the situation and behaviours. Asking questions, hypothesising, reality testing and evaluating are all activities closely linked to the concept of reflection. It is productive to 'replay' interactions in which we were involved. To picture oneself back in the situation and process what happened in some detail. For some people reflective writing is productive as a medium for the recording and analysis of interactions. The use of learning journals or communication diaries to record analytic and evaluative introspection are structures which may suit some people. Walker (1985) suggests that writing provides an objectivity and clarity to experiences by removing elements of subjective feeling that can obscure issues. These written records also provide data for further review in tutorials, supervision sessions or with peers. Some examples of reflective questions are given in Box 5.2.

Learning from feedback

Dickson et al (1989) discriminate between two types of feedback in relation to communication

skills. Intrinsic feedback is an integral feature of any interaction. Information is available from others involved during an interaction which indicates their responses to specific interventions. Learning to pay attention to intrinsic feedback during interactions and then responding accordingly is an important component of effective communication. Learning to concentrate sensitively on the cues and responses of the people with whom you are communicating helps in understanding the process of communication and informs the choice of response made. Extrinsic feedback refers to explicit information provided by others directly relating to the interactions. For example, a student on a placement contract might accompany his supervisor and focus particularly on his listening skills to observe and comment on an interaction with a client. The feedback in this case is supplementary to the actual interaction.

Both types of feedback are fundamental elements to improving communication skills. In the absence of extrinsic feedback the only perspective available is a subjective view which includes blind spots and limiting perceptions. Feedback serves the following functions:

- Promotion of self-awareness through the assimilation of information about how one is seen by others.
- Increase of options. More information provides new perspectives and different choices.
- Reinforcement. Positive feedback is likely to increase the frequency of productive behaviour.

Box 5.3 Principles of giving and receiving feedback

Giving feedback
1. Be specific. A clear statement of what precisely was observed is more helpful than a wide generalisation.
2. Achieve a balance. Highlight the strengths but also include aspects which require attention. Praise alone may make the person feel good but is not as helpful as balanced feedback.
3. Offer possible alternatives. Comment tentatively on how things could have been done differently. Avoid dogmatic advice.
4. Refer to behaviour rather than personal characteristics. Behaviour can be changed; personal characteristics cannot.
5. If a contract exists, stay within its boundaries i.e. if specific feedback is requested then this should be the focus of your comments.
6. Think what your feedback says about you.

Receiving feedback
1. Have an open mind. Avoid becoming defensive or argumentative and do not reject the feedback.
2. Ask for clarification.
3. Listen, consider and decide what you will do in the light of the feedback.

- Encouragement and motivation. A working culture which incorporates feedback tends to result in employees feeling more valued.

Providing feedback to others is in itself a communication skill and as such may be delivered constructively or destructively. Constructive feedback results in the four outcomes stated above. Destructive feedback leaves the recipient feeling negative and unclear about how to improve matters. Learning to provide constructive feedback adds value to the learning process but also has application in most other human interactions. The principles shown in Box 5.3 apply to the giving and receiving of constructive, extrinsic feedback.

INTERPERSONAL SKILLS TRAINING

Learning any skill requires progression through a number of different stages from identifying an individual skill through to the eventual mastery and integration of that skill. These stages are described by Egan (1985) and Dickson et al (1989). The following stages represent a training process which is an amalgamation of both descriptions.

Identification of individual non-verbal and verbal microskills appropriate to the context of the communication. This stage results in clarity of understanding of *what the skills are* in terms of definitions, behaviours, aims and application. It is achieved through reading, lectures, discussions.

Knowledge of how to use the skills. This is achieved by observing demonstrations of others using the skills. This may take the form of live demonstration, video or audio tapes. This stage facilitates progression from conceptual understanding to behavioural understanding.

Practice of the skills. The opportunity to try using the skills with peers in structured training sessions either using role play or preferably 'live' issues.

Evaluation of the practice through focused feedback. This stage enables reflection on one's own performance and also constructive feedback from peers and teachers. The intention is to confirm what is done well and correct what is not. A common structure is for a peer to observe the interaction and notice specifically what takes place.

Evaluation of the training process. Periodic evaluation of one's overall progress and the experience of the training process is useful in consolidating different experiences.

Implementation in the 'real world'. Putting the skills together within a nursing context is the final stage. Moving from the formalised learning environment to the practice setting and gradually integrating what has been learned so that it becomes second nature. This process is made easier by effective supervision, introspective reflection and feedback mechanisms.

A common experience of this learning process is to feel de-skilled at different stages. Often nurses feel discouraged by this temporary sense of incompetence.

The hypothetical dialogue in Box 5.4 is between a teacher and a student of the Diploma in Nursing Course Common Foundation programme, currently studying for a communication and interpersonal skills module. It illustrates some of the potential difficulties.

Box 5.4 The potential difficulties of interpersonal skills training

Student: 'I don't see the purpose of all this time we spend on learning communication skills. I can already communicate. I do it everyday with people. Surely there are more worthwhile subjects on which we could spend this time.'
Teacher: 'I appreciate that you already communicate at a sophisticated level and I hope that the work you are doing here is an acknowledgement of that. The emphasis that is placed on communication in the curriculum is based on the belief that nursing is essentially an interpersonal process and that we can all become more effective than we are right now. What do you think?'
Student: 'I think that we pick up communication as we go through life. If I have to stop to think about everything that I do and say I will be unable to do anything.'
Teacher: 'Unfortunately there is some truth in that. Learning interpersonal skills is difficult precisely because we have to focus on the complex details that we normally do not think about. Paradoxically this can make us feel less effective than when we just get on with it.'
Student: 'So what's the point?'
Teacher: 'The point is that this feeling of being de-skilled is only a temporary step on the learning curve. To use an analogy; when you drive your car you are performing extremely complex behaviours, judgements and reactions. The surprising fact is that you are rarely consciously thinking about how you will change gear, steer, use the accelerator and brakes etc. Somehow you just do it! If you have a passenger with you it is even possible to hold a conversation at the same time as carrying out these functions. Let's say that one day you decide to take advanced driving lessons. Your instructor prompts you to notice aspects of your driving performance by bringing them to your attention. This feels strange almost to the point that you feel you are unable to drive the car at all. Somehow the process has become laboured and disjointed just like it was when you first learned to drive. The feedback from the instructor leads you to do things differently and gradually the activity of driving becomes a different experience again. You become more aware of your strengths as a driver and of the areas you have to work at. Over time you become less clumsy and realise that you have refined skills and corrected bad practices of which you were previously not even aware. Eventually the whole process becomes a smooth concerted performance again but you now know that you are a better driver.'
Student: 'So what you are saying is that we will probably get worse before we get better at communication.'
Teacher: 'This is likely to be how you will experience this part of the course. Being asked to think more deeply about how you communicate is an unusual request but is necessary if you are to ultimately improve your communication with others.'

The learning curve represents a journey. At the beginning of the journey in Box 5.4 the nurse is communicating without thinking too deeply about it. The next step involves thinking about how he communicates but also feeling de-skilled. This is followed by a growing sense of competence which still requires much concentration. Finally, the nurse is able to communicate more competently without having to think so consciously about what he is doing.

A KNOWLEDGE OF PRAGMATIC THEORIES

Knowledge of a pragmatic theory of communication enables nurses to conceptualise what they are doing and provides a means to discuss interactions.

Two such theories which serve the purpose well are transactional analysis (Berne 1966) and six category intervention analysis (Heron 1990). The rationale for selecting these examples is that they are exhaustive in the sense that they may be applied to all interpersonal interactions in which nurses are likely to be involved during the course of their work.

Transactional analysis

Transactional analysis (TA) is much more than a framework for the analysis of interactions. It is also a theory of personality and a psychotherapeutic approach. The strengths of the theory lie in robust but simple concepts and their wide application to human encounters. A comprehensive description of the theory is beyond the scope of this text but students are advised to read from the reference section at the end of this chapter for further information.

The main concept of transactional analysis is the ego state. At any one time people manifest a part of their personality in a consistent pattern of behaviour, thoughts and feelings. These distinct patterns are known as ego states.

The three main ego states are indicated in Figure 5.3. The parent ego state refers to when a person behaves, thinks and feels in ways which are copied from his own parents or parental

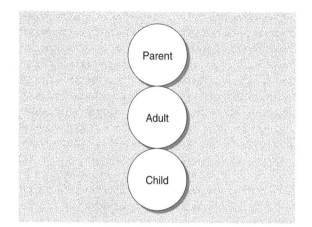

Figure 5.3 The three main ego states

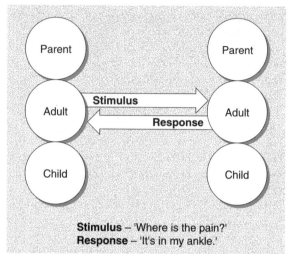

Stimulus – 'Where is the pain?'
Response – 'It's in my ankle.'

Figure 5.4 Adult to adult complementary transaction

figures. The child ego state refers to a pattern of behaviour, thoughts and feelings which are replayed from one's childhood. The adult ego state refers to behaviours, thoughts and feelings which are direct and appropriate responses to the here and now. None of the ego states have anything to do with time or whether one actually is a parent, adult or child. Young children at play often behave and relate to each other as if one were the parent and the other a child. Similarly, adults sometimes behave as children. Stewart & Joines (1987) suggest that a healthy and balanced personality requires all three of these ego states: 'adult' to enable problem solving, 'parent' to cope with society and its rules, 'child' for access to spontaneity, creativity and intuition. At any time one of the three ego states usually predominates.

This model provides a useful framework for understanding human interactions. Whenever two people are communicating with each other they are doing so from one of the three ego states. To observe and listen to them it is possible to discriminate between the different ego states and to note shifts that occur. Conceptually there is a way of analysing interactions. A transaction involves a stimulus and a response.

An example of an adult-to-adult complementary transaction is shown in Figure 5.4. The stimulus is a fact-finding question which invites a response from the adult ego state, which answers the question. Complementary transactions refer to those exchanges in which the arrows are

parallel and in which the ego state that is addressed is the one that responds. A second example of a complementary transaction involving different ego states is seen in Figure 5.5. The arrows remain parallel.

When transactions are complementary conversation tends to flow back and forth in a consistent manner. If, however, the arrows are crossed rather than parallel in a transaction then there is usually an interruption in communication while indivi-duals shift ego states (see Fig. 5.6).

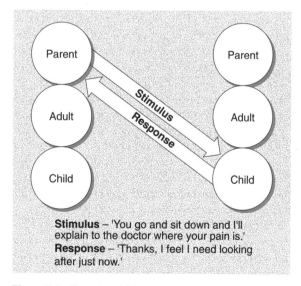

Stimulus – 'You go and sit down and I'll explain to the doctor where your pain is.'
Response – 'Thanks, I feel I need looking after just now.'

Figure 5.5 Parent to child complementary transaction

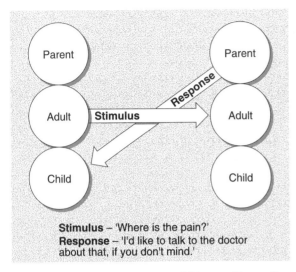

Stimulus – 'Where is the pain?'
Response – 'I'd like to talk to the doctor about that, if you don't mind.'

Figure 5.6 Adult-to-adult, parent to child crossed transaction

The example of a crossed transaction shows what happens when the ego state which is addressed is not the one which responds. There is usually a feeling of surprise when this happens. The response invites the other person to move into the child ego state, perhaps feeling put down and hurt. An understanding of this analytical framework provides the language and concepts to make sense of everyday interactions. Without such a framework communication is often difficult to process in a coherent manner. Also, the ego state model provides choices for the communicator. Where a language exists to describe what is happening there is more likelihood of seeing alternatives that are available during interactions. In this sense the model provides a structure for retrospective analysis and for informing future goal-directed communication.

Six category intervention analysis

Heron (1990 p. 7) claims six category intervention analysis to be 'exhaustive of the major sorts of valid interventions any practitioner needs to make in relation to clients'.

For nurses, this provides a very useful framework in which to examine their interactions with other people. Just as with transactional analysis, this model offers a conceptual structure to both assist the processing and to inform the

choices in nursing communication. The rationale for the inclusion of two such theories is to make the point that each is valid. There is no single complete and authoritative approach to examining such a complex activity as communication. Neither theory is 'real' but together they do provide alternative conceptual binoculars through which to view the world of communication.

Heron has identified six independent categories to classify the different types of interventions. He describes an intervention as 'any identifiable piece of verbal and/or non-verbal behaviour that is part of the practitioner's service to the client' (Heron 1990 p.3). The categories are shown in Figure 5.7 and are briefly described below.

The authoritative interventions are more directive categories in the sense that the nurse takes responsibility for the client. The facilitative categories are concerned with enabling clients to take responsibility for themselves. It is the context which determines the appropriate category to use. Heron (1990) regards each of the categories as equally valid as long as they are matched to the nurse's role, the client's needs and the purpose of the intervention. Each category includes specific skills and strategies which in turn require competent delivery:

- Prescriptive interventions include communication which aims to direct the other's behaviour, such as delegating tasks to colleagues or advising a client about taking medication.
- Informative interventions refer to interactions intended to give information, knowledge or meaning. Information is different to advice in that it tends to be more neutral and factual and less socially influencing, for example, explaining about a particular clinical procedure.

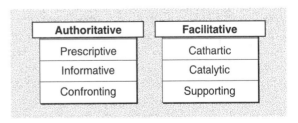

Figure 5.7 Six category intervention analysis (Heron 1990)

- Confronting interventions serve the purpose of challenging limiting perspectives, attitudes or behaviours, such as pointing out in a sensitive manner a client's self-defeating pattern of behaviour.
- Cathartic interventions enable others to express their emotions. Encouraging bereaved relatives to express the feelings associated with their loss is a case in point.
- Catalytic interventions help to draw out information and promote self-discovery and understanding.
- Supportive interventions affirm the worth of others and demonstrate respect and acceptance. Using counselling skills or running a support group are examples of this.

The strength of this framework is that it prompts nurses to be clear about the purpose of any communication in which they are involved. One way of thinking about the interventions is to compare them to playing a game of cards (see Box 5.5).

The skilled communicator is proficient in all six of the categories and able to move from one to another as the situation requires. Burnard & Morrison (1991) have conducted a number of studies of nurses' self-evaluation of skills using six category intervention analysis. The findings consistently suggest that nurses evaluate themselves as more skilled in the prescriptive,

informative and supportive categories and less skilled in the cathartic, catalytic and confronting categories. A number of possible reasons are suggested for this by the researchers but it may well be that these categories require more attention than they currently receive in nursing curricula.

In summary, knowledge of theoretical frameworks facilitates the analysis of communication. It also helps to clarify the purpose of specific interactions. Transactional analysis and six category intervention analysis are examples of theories which have wide application to nursing communication. Both theories serve to simplify analysis and reflection without omitting important issues.

THE PURPOSE OF THE INTERACTION

Whatever the context, a nurse's role is multi-faceted. Each facet of the role carries expectations on the part of the nurse and the others involved. The art of nursing is being sensitive to what is required in different situations and responding accordingly. Theories such as six category intervention analysis and transactional analysis are helpful in gaining clarity of the purpose and process of interactions. They are not, however, the full story. The nurse requires the interpersonal skills needed to ascertain data and information and to make a competent response. The other important element is less tangible but involves the ability to build a relationship with others based on sensitivity and understanding (these ideas are discussed in some detail in Chapter 9). When these three elements are integrated into nursing interactions the purpose and consequently the appropriate intervention will emerge.

Box 5.5 Six category intervention analysis at work

David is an experienced nurse who works on a children's ward. As he goes about his work he is approached by many different people during a shift. His experience, skills and education help him to choose appropriately how to respond to each encounter. If you were to observe him using six category intervention analysis you would notice how he advises parents about providing care at home; gives information to children in a way that they can understand; confronts a particularly boisterous youngster about his behaviour which is upsetting other children; encourages parents to express their fears about an operation; prompts a child to describe his situation during an assessment; and takes time to show his appreciation to his colleagues for their hard work. What makes David effective in his role is his ability to match skilled responses to the respective situations.

OVERVIEW

The potential for communication to go astray in nursing interactions is great. This has serious implications for all nurses because nursing is essentially an interpersonal process. Research over the last two decades has drawn attention to the importance of effective communication and has promoted the prominence of communication in nursing curricula. This chapter has highlighted some of the problems associated with nursing communication and suggested some solutions to improve matters. Becoming more effective as a communicator is a process of constant self-development.

This self-development involves several important strands which are detailed in Box 5.6.

Box 5.6   Four strands of self-development

1. Exploiting opportunities to increase awareness of oneself in an attempt to understand others and their experience of us.
2. Learning to use interpersonal skills in a competent, concerted and integrative fashion.
3. Referring to relevant theories in an attempt to analyse, reflect and process interactions.
4. Being clear about the purpose of interactions and matching interventions intentionally.

Combined, these strands can increase the chances that communication will be effective.

REFERENCES

Berne E 1966 Transactional analysis in psychotherapy. Grove Press, New York.

Boud D, Keogh R, Walker D 1985 Reflection: turning experience into learning. Kogan Page, London.

Burnard P 1985 Learning human skills: a guide for nurses. Heinemann, London.

Burnard P, Morrison P 1991 Nurses' interpersonal skills. Nurse Education Today, 11. 24—29

Dickson D A, Hargie O, Morrow N C 1989 Communication skills training for health professionals: an instructor's handbook. Chapman & Hall, London.

Dunn B 1991 Communication interaction skills. Senior Nurse, vol. 11, No 4. pp. 4—8.

Egan G 1985 Exercises in helping skills. A training manual to accompany the skilled helper, 3rd edn. Belmont, Brooks/Cole.

Egan G 1990 The skilled helper: a systematic approach to effective helping. Pacific Grove, Brooks/Cole.

Faulkner A 1985 The organisational context of interpersonal skills in nursing. In: C Kagan (ed) Interpersonal skills in nursing. Croom Helm, London.

Hayward J 1975 Information—a prescription against pain. The study of nursing care project reports. Series 2. No 5. London, Royal College of Nursing.

Heron J 1990 Helping the client. A creative practical guide. Sage, London.

Kemmis S 1985 Action research and the politics of reflection. In: Boud D, Keogh R, Walker D (eds) Reflection: turning experience into learning. Kogan Page, London, pp. 139—163.

Ley P 1988 Communication with patients—improving patient satisfaction and compliance. Croom Helm, London.

Macleod-Clark J 1984 Verbal communication in nursing. In: A Faulkner (ed) Recent advances in nursing 7: communication. Churchill Livingstone, Edinburgh.

Menzies E P 1970 The functioning of social systems as a defence against anxiety. Tavistock, London.

Patterson C H 1988 The function of automaticity in counsellor information processing. Counsellor, Education & Supervision, 27 pp. 195—202.

Peplau H 1988 Interpersonal relations in nursing. Macmillan, Basingstoke.

Rogers C 1967 On becoming a person. A therapist's view of psychotherapy. Constable, London.

Schon D A 1983 The reflective practitioner: how professionals think in action. Temple Smith, London.

Stein-Parbury J 1993 Patient and person. Developing interpersonal skills in nursing. Churchill Livingstone, Melbourne.

Stewart I, Joines V 1987 TA today: a new introduction to transactional analysis. Lifespace, Nottingham.

Stockwell F 1972 The unpopular patient: the study of nursing care project reports. Series 1. No.2. Royal College of Nursing, London.

Walker D 1985 Writing and reflection. In: Boud D, Keogh R, Walker D (eds) Reflection: turning experience into learning. Kogan Page, London.

CONTENTS

6

Communicating in groups

Robert J. Gates

INTRODUCTION

Previous chapters have concentrated on defining and exploring communication and describing how communication skills can be improved. The focus of this chapter is on communication in groups.

Nurses belong to both professional and non-professional groups, for example, family, hobby and interest-related, and staff organisational groups. Groups, therefore, are an integral part of their daily lives. Group communication is real and is a daily experience for most people. It is therefore common for most people, including nurses, to fail to acknowledge the complexity of groups and group communication. It is also because nurses may perceive groups as unproblematic that the study of this aspect of communication is so important.

Readers of this book are likely to have their own unique impressions and experiences of belonging to groups. Whilst acknowledging the richness of such experiences, an objective and reflective exploration and discussion of different theoretical approaches can add considerably to our understanding of groups. In addition, the study of groups is important because nurses need to understand the dynamics of interactions within groups to be able to use groups effectively to improve patient care.

It is important to acknowledge that most professional groups need to interact with other professional groups. Evidently, nurses work within a variety of community and institutional health care settings and are required to work collaboratively with other health care professions

(U.K.C.C. 1992). For these reasons nurses have an incumbent responsibility to study and improve upon their group communication.

DEFINING GROUPS

The definition of a 'group' depends upon which theoretical orientation is adopted to explain the phenomenon. Groups can vary in size as well as in formality/informality, for example compare the formal board or committee with an ad hoc discussion group. In addition, some groups are relatively permanent and durable whilst others are temporary. Despite these seemingly conflicting attributes Hargreaves (1975) has suggested that most groups have the following characteristics:

1. Members are in face to face relationships.
2. There is more than one member.
3. Members have common goals or purposes.
4. Members are differentiated into a structure.
5. Members subscribe to a set of norms.

These characteristics appear common to all explorations and definitions concerning groups and are used to reinforce and underpin the particular focus within this chapter.

Having outlined the characteristics of groups it would be useful at this stage to attempt a definition of the word. The reader is asked to consider, in the light of his/her own experience of groups, the definition proposed in Box 6.1.

Given this definition, three examples of groups to which a student of nursing might belong could include:

- A student group
- A ward team
- A procedure committee

Box 6.1 A definition of a 'group'

A group may be defined as:
Two or more individuals interacting with one another for an identifiable purpose and who share at least one goal. The individuals concerned normally occupy roles and adhere to rules and norms implicitly or explicitly agreed between members.

How does the proposed definition correspond with the characteristics of any one of these three groups? In the case of the student group, clearly it comprises more than one individual. In addition, a goal of all the students, presumably, is to successfully pass their course. If the reader thinks about the student group to which (s)he belongs, (s)he may be able to identify roles for each of the group members, for example leader, pacifier and joker. Also, the student group will most likely have developed its own rules to govern the behaviour of its members.

Having outlined a definition of groups a further point to consider is the number of individuals required to form a group. The reader will be aware, from experience, that plurality of persons does not in itself constitute a group. Clearly an individual is not a group, but are two people a group in the same sense as 10 or 15 people? Luft (1984) pointed to a number of generalisations that could be made concerning the size of groups:

1. Cohesion between members of a large group is weaker than that of a smaller group.
2. Very small groups have the unique characteristic of closeness of feeling between members.
3. Large groups are inclined to be more mechanical and business-like.

Some commentators have argued that the debate concerning the size of groups is a fruitless one (Hare 1976). It is the ability of the group to be able to interact and not the size that is important. In sociology a distinction is made between two types of groups: primary and secondary groups.

Primary groups. These may be understood as a type of group whose members are able to interact in an intimate, emotional and personal way. Within such groups the interactive dynamics of cooperating, fighting, imitating, loving and helping can be seen. Examples of such groups may include families, neighbourhood, recreational and occupational groups.

Secondary groups. These may be understood as larger groups whose members interact in a more impersonal way. Such groups are less sentimental and more formal than primary groups. The number of people belonging to this type of group is high, resulting in reduced opportunity for developing or maintaining close physical contact. These groups often have a clearly defined hierarchy and might include, for example, the management team of a N.H.S. Trust or the Royal College of Nursing's Society for Learning Disability Nurses.

DIFFERING THEORETICAL ORIENTATIONS

The formal study of groups is a relatively new addition to the Social Sciences. Knowles & Knowles (1972) suggest that it is only the contemporary scholar who has studied the small group. Historically much academic work addressed itself to the 'more remote aspects of social organisation'.

Knowles & Knowles (1972) provide a useful historical analysis of the differing theoretical perspectives of groups. The formal study of groups appeared to commence during the early part of this century. At that time, a number of leading academics were particularly interested in the idea of social control within groups. This early work was conjectural and was challenged in the 1920s because it was concerned with small groups and was based upon sociological studies. Instead, an empirical approach to researching groups developed, representing the first large scale attempt at understanding social processes within groups. The interest in this approach lay in understanding the conditions under which an individual's motivation is most effectively developed. Also during the 1920s Freud contributed to the study of groups. He postulated a psychological phenomenon of unconscious motivating forces of cohesion and control that originated from the family group. During the 1930s, 1940s and 1950s new approaches and orientations to understanding groups were developed. These different approaches to understanding groups are now briefly outlined.

The field approach

The field theory approach to groups can be ascribed to the work of Kurt Lewin (1951). The theory originated from physics, and was concerned with fields and forces. Lewin suggested that just as in the science of physics there are fields and forces, so too these are present in groups. Lewin applied this idea to the study of groups in an attempt to understand the forces and variables that affect a group's behaviour. Imagine a force field surrounding us and affecting objects placed near to it, for example repelling some objects and attracting others. Lewin suggested that such forces operate in just the same way within groups, affecting the behaviour of the group. Clearly these forces do not originate from a magnet but from interpersonal factors. Lewin argued that the strength and direction of group behaviour should be observed, as it is in physics, and measured to enable social scientists to eventually develop laws to explain group behaviour.

The psychoanalytical approach

The focus of the psychoanalytical approach is on the emotional and unconscious dimensions of the group process and is based on careful analysis of recorded group activity. Almost exclusively this approach is evidenced by therapeutic groups and has been elaborated upon, amongst others, by Bach (1954), Scheidlinger (1952) and Foulkes & Anthony (1957).

Another important contributor to this orientation was Bion (1961) who was interested in understanding the unconscious patterns of group life. Paradoxically the psychoanalytic approach to groups arose out of psychoanalysis used first in the treatment of individuals with emotional problems and then in the treatment of individuals in groups. Hansen et al (1976) has suggested that typically such a psychoanalytical group would meet weekly for approximately one and a half hours. During this time members would interact with one another, sharing problems and interpreting each other's actions and words.

The sociometric approach

The sociometric approach focuses on the social aspects of group life and how the emotional and interpersonal relationships between and among group members can be measured. Moreno (1934) developed a methodology for such measurement—a sociometric test. This test is a careful measure of the self-reported relationships between group members applied to a range of situations (each individual is asked to choose or reject companions for a joint activity). These measurements are then used to develop a profile of the structure of interaction within the group. The reported relationships can then be diagrammatically presented to illustrate the strength of relationships between group members.

During more recent years Knowles & Knowles (1972) have identified three recurrent themes in the field of group dynamics:

1. There has been a rapid expansion of the study of group phenomena by social scientists.
2. There has been an explosive development in the literature concerning the study of groups especially in technical journals.
3. There has been an increased interest in training personnel in group dynamics.

If the reader wishes to pursue a more in-depth study of the different theoretical orientations to groups, an excellent summary can be found in Cartright & Zander (1968).

Apart from differing theoretical approaches, groups may also be studied from both an organisational and an individual perspective.

GROUPS FROM AN ORGANISATIONAL PERSPECTIVE

The study of groups is important to organisations because they represent a mediator for the accomplishment of tasks. Indeed Knowles & Knowles (1972) suggest that groups have always been important throughout history for human accomplishment. Handy (1985) identifies 10 major headings of organisational functions that groups can achieve:

1. Distribution of work.
2. Problem solving and decision making.
3. Information processing.
4. Information and idea collection.
5. Management and control of work.
6. Testing and ratifying decisions.
7. Coordination and liaison.
8. Increased commitment and involvement.
9. Negotiation or conflict resolution.
10. Inquiry into the past.

Activity 6.1

1. Reflect momentarily on the organisational functions of groups and consider how much of your time has been spent in groups attempting to achieve one of those functions.

2. Interview a ward sister, charge nurse or senior nurse and try to find out how much of his/her time is spent in groups attempting to achieve organisational functions.

These organisational functions are of central importance to an understanding of groups. Imagine how an organisation would achieve any of its functions without the use of groups. Forming people into groups clearly provides a medium for the accomplishment of tasks that are beyond the scope of an individual.

Within health care the use of groups is common and provides an opportunity for reaching consensus decisions and providing holistic care. For example in learning disability nursing the client and members of the multidisciplinary team work together in planning the care for an individual. It is difficult to imagine the role of the nurse being enacted without reference to a wider group of health care professionals. By way of contrast, forming people into groups does not always result in effective, efficient or economic decisions and actions. In order for this to be achieved the objectives and the purpose of the group, the organisation and the individual all need to be congruent with one another. It is likely that readers of this chapter will have endured many group meetings of dubious relevance and usefulness where neither organisational nor individual objectives have been achieved. The phrase concerning some group experiences which readily springs to mind is 'What a waste of time'. This is because the individual leaves the meeting without any of his personal needs being met.

GROUPS FROM AN INDIVIDUAL PERSPECTIVE

From an individual perspective the study of groups is also important because groups provide an opportunity for the fulfilment of needs. Maslow (1954) suggests that human needs may be thought of as being organised into a hierarchy (see Fig. 6.1).

This section concentrates upon meeting some psychological needs such as self-esteem and belonging, although physiological needs may also be met through groups. Maslow suggests that needs at the bottom of the pyramid in Figure 6.1 need first to be satisfied before an individual can seek to address needs higher up the pyramid.

Satisfying the psychological needs through group membership is important to the level of an individual's commitment to the group. If the goals of a group, and an organisation are incompatible with that of an individual, then group cohesion will fail. This may lead the group to become a non-productive unit, i.e. is a collection of individuals rather than a group.

Communication within groups can be dynamically linked to the fulfilment of needs. For example, an individual might use a group to satisfy the need of self-esteem. Knowles & Knowles (1972) have suggested that a person's internal facets of emotional tendencies, for example biological needs, experience, personal goals and beliefs, interact with the external dynamics of a group. This combination of group

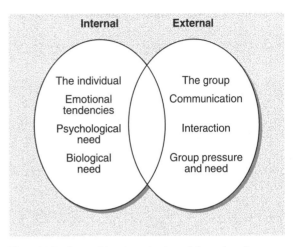

Figure 6.2 Internal facets and external dynamics of group communication

external forces and the individual's internal facets is an important concept. This is because the dynamics of interaction and communication within a group depend upon this interplay between the individual and the collective, i.e. the group, as demonstrated in Figure 6.2.

Handy (1985) has suggested that individuals use groups to:

1. Satisfy social needs.
2. Establish self-concept.
3. Give or receive support and help.
4. Share with others.

From an individual perspective it would appear that supportive, productive group encounters offer the potential to facilitate psychological need reduction. However, the mismatch between the individual need and group performance can lead to negative group experience. Such an experience may lead to individual needs not being met. In other words the meeting of individual needs is dependent upon the dynamics of and communication within groups.

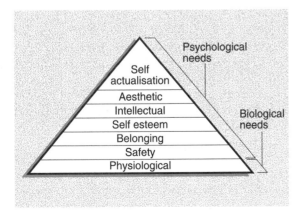

Figure 6.1 After Maslow's hierarchy of needs

Activity 6.2

Identify and reflect upon those groups to which you belong. Which of the needs identified by Maslow (1954) do you think are partially or completely met by those groups that you have identified?

GROUP INTERACTION

This section of the chapter explores in detail one approach to analysing the processes of interaction within groups, that of interaction analysis. However, this emphasis does not exclude the value or richness of other theoretical orientations which have been briefly described earlier in this chapter. The reader is strongly advised to study a variety of theoretical orientations to groups because wide reading and reflection will help nurses to make sense of their experience in groups.

INTERACTION ANALYSIS

A significant contributor to this approach is Bales (1950) who developed an interaction analysis system. Essentially this system consists of 12 categories of observable behaviour that can be recorded by a rater. The categories can be divided as follows:

- Three of the categories are occupied by social, emotional positive expressive acts of communication. These categories refer to constructive, helpful behaviours within a group.

- Six categories are instrumental and are used to record interaction concerned with the group completing a task. The instrumental categories are viewed as neutral acts of communication.
- The remaining three categories are occupied by social, emotional negative aspects of communication. These categories refer to destructive, unhelpful behaviours within a group.

See Figure 6.3 for a modified system.

Interaction analysis uses the observations of a rater(s) who categorises each act of communication within a group. Each of the 12 categories has equal weighting and refers to a single act of communication by a group member. The system requires the rater(s) to categorise both verbal and non-verbal communication within a group. This is achieved by attributing a number to each member of the group and then recording each act of communication within a single category. The direction of communication is recorded by placing the number of the originator of the interaction, over the number of the receiver. In Figure 6.3 group member 7 is shown offering an opinion to group member 5 during the sixth minute of interaction. The time interval for analysis is one minute. Thus at the completion of each minute the rater(s) proceed to categorising communication during the next time span, i.e. minute.

Categories	Minutes															Total
	1	2	3	4	5	6	7	8	9	10	11	12	13	14	15	
1 Seems friendly																
2 Reduces tension																
3 Agrees																
4 Offers suggestions																
5 Offers opinions						7/5										
6 Offers information																
7 Seeks information																
8 Seeks opinion																
9 Seeks suggestions																
10 Disagrees																
11 Appears tense																
12 Seems unfriendly																
Total																

Figure 6.3 A simplified interaction analysis recording sheet

During the exercise the rater(s) should adopt the role of generalised other, i.e. the rater(s) should attempt to experience the significance of the interaction, as if it had occurred to himself. The rater(s) should also attempt to categorise as many units of interaction as possible within each one minute interval. Experienced raters are capable of rating as many as 10 to 15 scores a minute. Clearly, however, the number of ratings will depend on the level of communication within the group.

A feature of the Bales' interaction analysis system is that there exists a high degree of inter-rater reliability. That is, if a number of raters were, independently but simultaneously, categorising the interaction of a group, their findings would be very similar. This is important if one wishes to obtain reliable data which may be used to decide how to improve the dynamics of a particular group. For an example, see the case history in Box 6.2.

Box 6.2 Case history

A group of nurses in a residential home for people with a learning disability were experiencing difficulty in reaching a decision about the management of care for a resident. This particular resident had very over-protective parents. The difficulties originated from the very different approaches that nurses were using to manage the situation when the parents seemingly interfered in the resident's care. When the issue was discussed at team meetings, the discussion repeatedly ended with heated exchanges between group members with no consensus, and therefore no resolution, of the situation. The home leader requested that a nurse colleague, experienced in group work, should come to the home to observe the group and recommend strategies to improve communication.

To provide the nurse with a stable and reliable database of interactive processes, a video recording was made of a group meeting. This recording facilitated the nurse in analysing the group processes on more than one occasion. Repeated analysis of data can improve the number of units of interaction analysed, therefore lending greater clarity to the processes of group interaction.

The seating arrangements of the group members were informal, however, there did exist certain constraints due to the position of the video camera, so that the whole group could be accommodated.

Case history analysis

Group analysis

From the recording of the case history outlined in Box 6.2, 15 minutes of analysis are provided here to help the reader gain insight into the dynamics of this particular group and into the use of this approach to studying group interaction. The 15 minutes are divided into three 5 minute phases, during which a total of 76 acts of communication were analysed. Of these 76 responses some 46 (61%) units of interaction occurred within phases one and two. Within phase three there were some 30 (39%) units of interaction recorded.

The total number of responses in the 'expressive positive' categories amounted to 10 (13%). Within the 'instrumental' categories there were 48 (63%) responses, and within the 'expressive negative' categories there were 18 (24%) responses.

The percentages for each category are provided in Figure 6.4 which shows that the greatest percentile score occurred within category 5, some 20% of the total interaction of the group. Second was category 7 which accounted for 18% of the

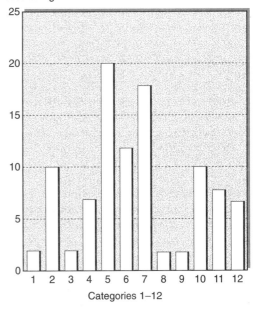

Percentages of used categories

Categories 1–12

Figure 6.4 % category analysis of group interaction

total interaction. Thus, nearly 40% of the group's interaction would appear to be concerned with the giving of opinion and the asking for orientation. Category 6 accounted for some 12% of the group's interaction and categories 2 and 10 represented equally 10%. Category 11 accounted for 8% and categories 4, 8 and 12 represented 7% each of the interactions recorded.

It can be seen from the group profile that categories 1, 3, 8 and 9 accounted for 8% of the group's interaction.

The location of the frequencies within the categories led the rater to an initial conclusion that the group had difficulty in evaluating comments between one another. This may have prevented the group from moving forward to achieve the group task. The high level of interaction in categories 5, 7, 10, 11 and 12, led the rater to conclude that there was a problem of effective communication between members and a difficulty in reducing tension within the group.

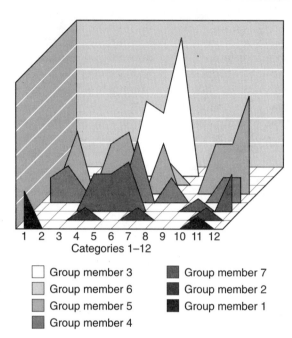

Categories 1–12

- Group member 3
- Group member 6
- Group member 5
- Group member 4
- Group member 7
- Group member 2
- Group member 1

Figure 6.5 Graphic representation of individual group members (not to scale)

Individual analysis

A superficial analysis of the group findings tells us little above that which we already knew. However, further analysis at individual level is possible, telling us about each individual's acts of communication and with whom this interaction took place.

Activity 6.3

The reader is asked to study Figure 6.5 and attempt to analyse how each individual interacted within each of the categories. Who was the most and least interactive?

Which individual was recorded as using the most negative interaction? The reader may like to refer to Table 6.1 to remind himself of the categories.

There were, in total, 7 individuals within the case history group and individual analysis of interaction provides interesting insights into the type of interactions that were occurring (see Fig. 6.5). In Activity 6.3, the reader might have made some if not all of the following observations:

- Group members 1, 2 and 6 contributed little to overall interaction within the group.

- Group member 3 contributed some 24% to the interaction within the group and was the second most 'interactive' individual. Overall, many of this individual's interactions occurred within the instrumental categories, particularly category 7. This may indicate an individual seeking to communicate effectively by frequently asking questions.

- Group member 4 contributed to 17% of the total interaction recorded and engaged in both expressive positive and expressive negative acts of interaction. 6% of interaction was spent using expressive positive acts of communication and 50% of the interaction took place in the instrumental categories.

- Group member 5 contributed some 35% to the overall acts of communication within the group. Over half of this interaction was engaged in expressive negative communication. This is significantly higher than the total number of expressive negative acts of communication by the remainder of the entire group. Only a small amount of the invididual's interaction was expressed positively.

• Group member 7 contributed to 14% of the interaction rated, of which 4% was engaged in expressive negative acts of communication whilst the remaining 10% of interaction took place within the instrumental categories 4, 5 and 6.

Conclusions from the exercise

The most interactive member of the group was member 5 and a significant component of her contribution to interaction was the use of expressive negative categories. When the rater analysed the pattern of interaction he found that 90% of this individual's negative interaction was directed at group member 3. Such a finding raised questions concerning the nature of the relationship between the two individuals and may have been indicative of two people not getting on. Gahagan (1975) offers another alternative by suggesting that early on within the time scale of a group encounter, time is spent engaging in a 'battle for the floor', by the highest contributors to the group.

This is interesting because group member number 3 was the next most interactive person in the group. However, it may have been no more sinister than Bales' (1953) suggestion that it is common for participation in groups to be unequal with one or two group members contributing more than others.

The findings from the analysis exercise were presented to the home leader and subsequently to the team of nurses but did not resolve the group tensions and difficulties. They did, however, provide group members with new and different insights into the ways in which they were communicating with each other. Also, the exercise paved the way for further group work with the team with a view to improving group effectiveness in decision making.

LEADERSHIP IN GROUPS

Most groups appear to have a leader who is either formally appointed, for example a chairperson, or who emerges as a leader because of some special skill or knowledge (an informal arrangement).

It is unusual to find the leader of a group totally dominating interaction, whether appointed formally or informally (Hargie et al 1981). Individual members of a group often emerge to provide acts of leadership when their unique expertise, knowledge or skills are required by the group. Baron et al (1992) make a distinction between task orientated leaders and people orientated leaders.

Task orientated leaders

This style of leader uses time effectively, sets clear priorities and frequently makes executive decisions. It is sometimes important for groups to have task orientated leaders especially when there is a need to focus on a task to resolve some problem promptly. An example of a task orientated leader may be a senior nurse appointed by the chief executive of an N.H.S. Trust to develop a policy for the administration of medicines. On calling a meeting the senior nurse clearly outlines the task set for the group and the short time scale in which the group must achieve its objectives. At subsequent meetings the senior nurse does not permit discussion on anything other than the task at hand. Once the policy is agreed between the members the group is disbanded.

People orientated leaders

This style of leader is more concerned with the feelings and problems of group members. The concern is for the person, rather than the task, and it is suggested that this type of leadership produces higher group morale. An example of a person orientated leader is a senior nurse, again appointed by the Chief Executive of an N.H.S. Trust but this time to set up a 'think tank' on how to reduce sickness and absenteeism amongst staff. The senior nurse believes it important to understand the reasons for sickness and absenteeism and so establishes a small group to discuss these issues. At all the meetings feelings and problems are openly discussed in an attempt by the senior nurse to fully appreciate the difficulties experienced by employees and to decide how the situation might best be managed. The group meetings are relaxed and the senior nurse constantly praises and reinforces group members for their contributions.

Student nurses will probably be able to reflect upon past group experiences where either one or both of these styles of leadership have been evident. 'One or both' is emphasised because it is unlikely that the exclusive use of purely one style of leadership is used without the other. In other words, it is the unique circumstances surrounding the group and its task or goals that possibly suggest the most relevant or productive style of leadership for any given group.

Consider the activity described below and attempt to identify which style of leadership would be the most appropriate and why. To help formulate an answer reflect on your own experience of successful group encounters and use this knowledge to guide your thinking.

Activity 6.4

A senior nurse manager has asked you to arrange a small group meeting of health care workers to discuss how to implement primary nursing on your ward. She has told you that she will give you her full support in this venture, as the ward team are renowned for their resistance to change. You have identified a group, agenda and venue for the first meeting and are now trying to decide which style of leadership would suit the group. Identify a leadership style and discuss the reasons for your choice with a colleague.

UNSPOKEN, UNCONSCIOUS GROUP INTERACTION

Having read the section on interaction analysis you may be forgiven for believing that it is possible to identify, classify and therefore analyse all interaction within groups. This is clearly not possible because of the many subtle, unspoken and unconscious interaction processes that occur and that cannot be measured. This unconscious and unspoken interaction arises from a mixture of individual experiences and the hidden agendas of some group members.

It is the individual's unconscious experience and knowledge of others that often leads the individual to develop theories about other people. For example a person who views others through

a behaviourist perspective may find his group behaviour to be shaped by these beliefs. A behaviourist believes in the importance of reinforcement to desired behaviour and, within a group situation, may deliberately reinforce submissive behaviour from others in order to dominate the direction of group interaction.

Sometimes an individual may take a 'hidden agenda' to a meeting, i.e. a set of desired outcomes which are not shared with other group members. The individual will then covertly attempt to manipulate the meeting and the behaviour of others to bring about a successful adoption of his desired outcomes. An example of this may be a staff nurse who does not want the ward team to adopt the new shift pattern, proposed by the ward manager, because it will significantly affect the child minding arrangement he has made. When the new shift pattern is discussed at the ward meeting the staff nurse identifies a range of problems likely to be experienced by patients and their relatives, should the shift pattern be introduced. Although this is a simplistic example it does demonstrates how group situations often contain unspoken factors that affect the dynamics of the group.

THE COMPLEXITY OF GROUPS WITHIN ORGANISATIONS

Having described interaction within groups, aspects of their complexity are now explored and applied to nursing practice.

GROUP COHESIVENESS

Zander (1981) defines the term cohesiveness as 'the resultant forces which are acting on the members to stay in the group'. Within groups where there is high cohesiveness, or strong forces acting upon members to stay together, a number of features appear prominent. These include good organisation, good relationships and a good record of achievement (see Box 6.3).

These features of cohesiveness are supported by research in this area. Seashore (1954) studied

Box 6.3 The features of a cohesive group	
Good organisation:	This factor refers to group members being clear about their role within the group. There is also evidence of effective interaction between group members. There is a feeling of good organisation of group activity and this leads members to feel comfortable and secure within the group.
Good relationships:	This factor is characterised by a free and easy exchange of interaction between group members and may be evidenced by a feeling of 'liking' between group members. This is what Dion et al (1978) refer to as the affective bonds between group members.
Good record of achievement:	The third feature of highly cohesive groups is the apparent ability to both undertake and successfully complete tasks ascribed to it.

cohesiveness in 228 industrial working groups. His study found that in groups where high cohesiveness was evident there was less anxiety, less variation in productivity and greater prestige attributed to members' own jobs. The implications for nursing here are important. Clearly, groups of health care professionals that can be helped to become more cohesive may, in effect, make a greater contribution to assigned tasks compared with groups with little cohesion. Cohesion is a term used to describe the mutual feeling of well being and 'pulling together' experienced by some groups. Readers, no doubt, will be able to recall positive group experiences when this feeling of cohesion was evident. Generally such experiences are remembered because individuals believe that a group was well organised, that tasks were achieved and that members grew to like one another. In other words the experience of highly cohesive groups is generally a favourable one. It is important here to reaffirm the importance of understanding the necessity to meet individual needs and the way in which this affects group dynamics (see p. 75).

GROUP PRESSURES AND NORMS

Given the definition of groups offered earlier, of central relevance to this section are the issues of 'sharing at least one goal and adhering to group rules and norms'.

Clearly if a group member moves away from the goals of the group then they also move away from being a member of the group. This may be evidenced in dramatic terms, when an individual feels that he no longer shares sufficient commonalty with a group to justify his continued membership and so resigns from the group. Alternatively, the group may seek to reject the individual on the basis that he no longer demonstrates loyalty to the group. An example of this may be a student of nursing who refuses to support his fellow students in a group when complaining about the quality of lectures by a nurse tutor.

More frequently, when an individual group member has difficulty in agreeing to the goals, and/or conforming to the rules and norms of the group, he experiences strong pressures to conform. The studies of Sheriff (1935), Asch (1955) and Milgram (1963) demonstrate the strength and pressure of the group processes that are used to bring about conformity from the individual. Failure to conform will initially lead to marginalisation, but if the differences between the individual and the group persist or deepen then inevitably the non-conforming individual must, or will be asked to leave the group.

With the increasing use of multidisciplinary teams to reach consensus decisions concerning the management of patient care, it is important for nurses to be aware of the need to work constructively within groups whilst ensuring that they do not succumb to group pressure for inappropriate care planning. Nurses must always demonstrate their invested concern for the caring ethic. This may sometimes lead to tensions between acting as an advocate for an individual on the one hand and conforming to group pressure on the other. Clearly such tensions and potential conflict may prove problematic both for the nursing practitioner and for group communication (Gates, 1994).

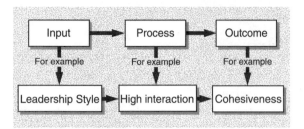

Figure 6.6 The relationship of input and process to group outcome (performance)

GROUP PERFORMANCE

Group performance must logically be preceded by an input and a process and these two variables have been shown to affect the performance, or outcome, of the group in the following ways.

Input. Factors known to affect the type of interaction in groups include: leadership styles, group member personality characteristics, group size, group history and lastly the type of task assigned to the group.

Process. Group interaction, as we have already discussed, can be analysed systematically. The results of such analysis seem to indicate that some groups are more effective than others. For example, groups that have a high recorded level of positive interaction appear to be highly cohesive.

Output (performance). This may be considered as a quantifiable measure of, for example, quality and speed of solution, group cohesiveness and attitude change.

The variables of input and process are discussed at length by Berkowitz (1978) who records a wealth of research data to support the interactive nature of the relationship between input and process and group output. The nature of this relationship is demonstrated in Figure 6.6 which shows how cohesiveness as an outcome is mediated through high interaction and is also related to leadership style.

GROUP RIVALRY AND ISOLATION

The last part of this section briefly considers group rivalry and isolationism. Within any large organisation groups have the potential to form rival relationships with other groups (Handy 1985). A subsequence of such rivalry may be a tendency for a particular group to isolate itself from the wider context of an organisation. Clearly, groups working in isolation, regardless of their performance, are of little use to the wider organisation and the meeting of patient need. Handy (1985) described in his book concerning organisations, the idea of differentiation. This term may be understood to represent the wide variety of people and groups who possess a plurality of skills and expertise. If these differing skills and expertise are not acknowledged, and somehow accommodated within an organisation, then there is the potential for the differentiated environment to 'tear itself apart or fail to communicate at all' (Handy 1985).

Clearly the range of health care settings in which nurses work represent complex organisational structures, with a plethora of professional groups with the potential for both rivalry and isolationism. This is because the many different professional groups perceive themselves as different in some way from other groups within a hospital or community setting. Nowhere are such difficulties better expressed than by The Audit Commission (1992) who identify a number of problems in primary health care concerning the use of teams. They say:

Multidisciplinary working, particularly within primary health teams, is also difficult. Separate lines of control, different payment systems leading to suspicion over motives, diverse objectives, professional barriers and perceived inequalities in status, all play a part in limiting the potential of multi-professional, multi-agency teamwork. These undercurrents often lead to rigidity within teams with members adhering to narrow definitions of their roles and preventing the creative and flexible responses required to meet the variety of human need presented. They are also likely to lead to lower morale. For those working under such circumstances efficient teamwork remains an elusive ideal.

(The Audit Commission 1992)

The use of multidisciplinary teams is something that nurses have advocated for many years and clearly represent a potential medium for the reduction of professional inter-group tension. However, their use must not be seen as unproblematic. In relation to the nature of relationships between doctors and nurses, for example Mackay (1993) observes that 'the extent to which doctors and nurses manage to work together affects patients' experiences. Inter-professional relations are not some esoteric aspect of health care. They should centrally inform the way in which patients are treated and cared for.'

The need to surface, discuss and work through tensions within a team may well be required before the team begins to function as an effective group. This is achieved by effective group communication.

THE NURSE AND EFFECTIVE GROUP COMMUNICATION

The last two sections of this chapter look at how the nurse can apply his knowledge and unique experience of groups to situations encountered in practice.

ANALYSING ONE'S OWN CONTRIBUTION

Earlier within this chapter we looked at interaction analysis and how it could be used to observe individual contributions within a group. Here we briefly explore the ways in which nurses may analyse their own contributions to group communication.

In keeping with one of the underlying beliefs of this book a process of reflection is advocated. The familiarity of the experience of belonging to a group may lead to behaviours within groups becoming habitualised. This concept is explored by Berger & Luckman (1967) who suggest that when human action is repeated many times, there is the potential for those actions to be taken for granted. Chapters 7, 8 and 9 emphasise the need for practitioners to reflect upon their practice. Jervis (1992) explores reflective practice in nursing and makes an important distinction between this and thoughtful practice (see Box 6.4).

Thoughtful and/or reflective practice may be useful in attempting to analyse one's own contribution to group communication during

Box 6.4	The difference between thoughtful and reflective practice
Thoughtful practice	Thoughtful practice is characterised by actions which are consciously monitored by actors (nurses) during practice. Thoughtful practice within a group context, refers to an individual monitoring and evaluating his own communication and the outcome of each interaction. Whilst providing nursing care a nurse practitioner should identify whether outcomes have materialised as planned and, if not, retrospection should occur. The processes of retrospection will help the practitioner to identify why the outcomes have not been achieved. Thoughtful practice is a 'here and now' learning experience. It is a form of reflection that occurs during, not after, practice.
Reflective practice	Reflective practice, by way of contrast, is learning from questions posed in 'taken for granted' situations. Jervis (1992) believes reflective practice to start at the point where such questioning begins. The process of reflective practice may be self-induced or other induced (Jervis 1992). Reflective practice, therefore, is qualitatively different from thoughtful practice and may be operationalised by contemplation, reflective skills and experimental knowledge. It seeks to pursue and use 'good theory' in practice. An example of reflective practice may be thinking deeply about the merits, or otherwise, of taking routine clinical observations such as blood pressure.

and/or after each interaction. Nurses could consider their effect upon group communication by asking the sort of questions listed below:

- How did I help communication within the group?
- Did I contribute to resolving the task set for the group?
- Did I engage in negative expressive acts of communication and if I did, what effect did these have upon interaction?
- How can I learn from my experience to improve my contribution to communication within groups?

GROUP PROBLEM SOLVING

A positive attribute of a group is its ability to resolve problems that are possibly too complex for an individual to resolve by himself. Smith & Bass (1982) identify two types of group that are used in problem solving: the committee/decision making group and the brain storming group.

The committee/decision making group. Usually such groups are appointed by managers to resolve a specific problem and/or provide long-standing advice and analysis on a specialist area. Generally committees such as these can be quite formal with the appointment of a chairperson and secretary and the taking of minutes or notes.

The brain storming group. This type of group is usually convened to generate great numbers of ideas to provide fast and possibly new insights into solving or rethinking a problem. The varied and individualistic background of group members provides a rich resource for the achievement of the group task. Priestly et al (1978) identified four basic rules governing the conduct of brain storming sessions.

1. Judgements concerning ideas generated must not be made until the exercise has finished.
2. The group should concern itself with producing a vast quantity of ideas rather than worrying about the quality of the ideas.
3. Group members should allow themselves to think freely; this is thought to facilitate creativity.
4. Ideas offered by one group member should be built upon and developed by other group members.

In both these types of group the problem solving approach used incorporates the following three stages:

- Clarifying the task to be completed.
- Identifying solutions.
- Developing and implementing action plans.

These three stages are critical to effective problem solving within groups. Clearly communication between individual group members will have a significant impact upon the ability to resolve a problem.

IMPLICATIONS FOR PRACTICE

MANAGING A GROUP

To manage a group requires considerable skills in the management of people, as well as the ability to communicate effectively. Equally important are the skills of motivating individuals and using resources effectively.

This section can do no more than focus upon some aspects of communication related to the management of groups. Those aspects described can be applied to formal primary groups for example, a ward meeting in a district general hospital, or to informal primary groups such as an impromptu community learning disability team gathering.

The management of groups can be divided into three main areas of consideration, each of which is discussed below.

Group leadership

The pursuit of a single style of leadership may not always be productive in achieving a task set for a group. Therefore, the leader of any group must firstly attempt to determine which particular leadership style is the most pertinent to the task at hand. This frequently results in the leader adopting an eclectic style, based upon both people and task centred approaches. Whether single or eclectic styles of leadership are adopted, it is important that the leader of the group is able to facilitate interaction within the group. Such facilitation, whilst being a demanding role, is crucial to a feeling of well being, both to the individual and the group as a whole in its performance. Another enabling role of the leader is that of helping members 'see a way through'. Often groups experience ambiguity concerning tasks ascribed to them. This ambiguity can lead to confusion, negativity and disaffection. Lastly an important role for the leader is to prevent group members from getting 'bogged down' and helping them to focus on the task and its accomplishment.

Group environment

The physical environment in which a group operates is important to its processes and outcomes. Factors which are conducive to the well being of individuals, and which contribute to effective communication, within groups include:

- A warm, comfortable and well ventilated room in which to work. It is important that the environment chosen for the group is relatively free from interruption.
- The opportunity for members of the group to be able to obtain satisfactory refreshments and access to toilet facilities is obviously important. These factors need to be considered alongside breaks in the group's activities. Interaction within groups can become stale and non-productive if members are not permitted to break away from very focused task solving exercises.

Whilst these environmental factors might appear trivial they are extremely important to group members. The reader is asked to reflect again on discussion earlier within the chapter concerning individual need. If the leader of a group fails to acknowledge the importance of meeting physical and psychological need, then this may adversely affect the life and productivity of the group.

Group dynamics

The manner in which a group leader facilitates interaction within a group often contributes significantly to the dynamics of the group. It is important for the leader of a group not only to encourage evaluation of an individual group member's contribution, but to ensure that evaluative comments are constructive and not destructive. The group leader must also attempt to encourage all members of the group to listen to one another. A difficult task for a group leader is the encouragement of quieter group members. Often one or two members feel intimated by other members and therefore their contribution is not forthcoming. Lastly, an important role of the leader is to recognise tensions within the group

and if necessary deal appropriately with negative group members.

Poulton & West (1993) identify a number of characteristics that a group leader might find useful in the management of groups, especially where these may be multidisciplinary. These include:

- Identifying a common objective or goal either for, or with, the group to which all the group members agree to work to.
- Establishing a clear understanding of each person's role in the group.
- Establishing a mutual respect for the role of each member of the group.

Handling negative group members

Earlier within the chapter the reader was introduced to a case history concerning problem-atic communication within a group (see Box 6.2). The difficulty experienced by the group during the period of analysis appeared to be located with one individual and the nature of his negative interactions, particularly with one other group member. It is not unusual for nurses, or indeed any group member, to encounter negative group members. This section considers how a nurse could manage such individuals, encouraging them to become constructive members of a group rather than negative ones. This is important to nurses for two major reasons:

- First, identifying and resolving the problem of negative individuals within groups helps to improve group performance.
- Second, but equally important, is the issue of personal group experience. If an individual's experience within a group is that it is a 'waste of time' this is usually because of group problems, often due to negative group members. Failure to identify and resolve such problems allows the status quo to continue unchallenged.

Smith & Bass (1982) identify a number of strategies that a nurse could use constructively as a group leader to help a negative group member become a positive contributor. These strategies include:

- Creating a feeling of belonging.
- Creating a sensitive environment.
- Encouraging participation and contribution.
- Valuing diverse opinion.
- Creating a sense of commitment.

These strategies are worthy of further discussion. Firstly, it is important to note that all the strategies identified can be adopted by a nurse in groups to which they are contributing as members, or groups that they may lead. Group experience sometimes leaves an individual feeling isolated. This may occur for a number of reasons, as has already been outlined in the section on group pressures and norms. The feeling of belonging is a psychological need for all individuals that can be met by belonging to a group. A nurse can help meet this need by ensuring that the contributions and participation of all individuals are valued. This requires all group members to contribute to the creation of a friendly and supportive environment. This also means that individual alternative view points to group decisions should be discussed openly and not rejected on a personal basis. Valuing the contributions and participation of all members fosters a climate in which the negative group member may develop a feeling of belonging. Equally important is that such a climate may well

prevent the development of negative group members in the first instance.

It is an unfortunate but inescapable fact, however, that some individuals fail, despite help, to constructively contribute to the life of the group. When this occurs it may be important to remove such an individual from the group.

CONCLUSION

Within this chapter the author has introduced the reader to a definition of groups as well as exploring different types of group and differing theoretical orientations concerning the study of groups. Emphasis has been placed upon one approach to analysing interaction within groups, using an interaction analysis system. By way of contrast, it has been acknowledged that there are other equally valid, rich and insightful ways of analysing and understanding interaction within groups. Lastly the author has attempted to demonstrate how the reader's own knowledge of groups can be synthesised with both the theory and research into groups and applied to the practice of nursing.

It is hoped that this chapter has created, within the reader, a desire to further explore, reflect upon and move toward a richer understanding of communication in groups.

REFERENCES

Audit Commission 1992 Homeward bound: a new course for community health. H.M.S.O. London.
Asch S 1955 Opinions and social pressure. Scientific American 193, 31–55.
Bach G R 1954 Intensive group psychotherapy. Ronald, New York.
Bales R 1950 Interaction process analysis: a method for the study of small groups. Addison-Wesley, Massachusetts.
Baron R S, Kerr N, Miller N 1992 Group process, group decision, group action. Open University Press, Buckingham.
Berger P, Luckmann T 1967 The social construction of reality. Penguin, London.
Berkowitz L (ed) 1978 Group processes. Academic Press, New York.
Bion W R 1961 Experiences in groups, 2nd edn. Basic Books, New York.
Cartright W D, Zander A F 1968 Group dynamics: research and theory, 3rd edn. Tavistock, London.
Dion K L, Baron R S, Miller N 1970 Why do groups make riskier decisions than individuals? In: Berkowitz (ed)

Advances in experimental social psychology. Vol. 5, 306–77.
Foulkes S H, Anthony E J 1957 Group psychotherapy: the psychoanalytic approach. Penguin Books, London.
Gahagan J 1975 Interpersonal and group behaviour. Methuen, London.
Gates B 1994 Advocacy: a nurse's guide. Scutari Press, London.
Handy C 1985 Understanding organisations, 3rd edn. Penguin, London.
Hansen J C, Warner R W, Smith E M 1976 Group counselling: theory and process. Rand McNally Pub. Co., Chicago.
Hare A O 1982 Creativity in small groups. Sage, London.
Hargie O, Saunders C, Dickson D 1981 Social skills in interpersonal communication, 2nd edn. Croom Helm, London.
Hargreaves D 1975 Interpersonal relations and education. Stu. edn. Routledge & Kegan Paul, London.
Jervis P 1992 Reflective practice and nursing. Nurse Education Today. 12, 174–181.
Knowles M L, Knowles H 1972 Introduction to group dynamics. Follet Pub. Co.

Lewin K 1951 Field theory in social science. Harper, New York.

Luft J 1984 Group processes: an introduction to group dynamics, 3rd. edn. Mayfield Publishing Company, California.

Mackay L 1993 Conflicts in care, medicine and nursing. Chapman & Hall, London.

Maslow A 1954 Motivation and personality, 2nd edn. Harper & Row, New York.

Milgram S 1974 Obedience to authority. Harper & Row, New York.

Moreno J L 1934 Who shall survive? Nervous and Mental Diseases Publishing Co., Washington.

Poulton B C, West M A 1993 Effective multidisciplinary teamwork in primary health care. Journal of Advanced Nursing. 18, 918–925.

Priestly P, McGuire J, Flegg D, Hemsley V, Welham D 1978 Social skills and personal problem solving: a handbook of methods. Tavistock Publications, London.

Scheidlinger S 1952 Psychoanalysis and group behaviour. Norton, New York.

Seashore S E 1954 Group cohesiveness in the individual work group. Ann Arbor Pub, University of Michigan.

Sheriff M 1935 A study of some social factors in perception. Archives of psychology. 27, No. 187.

Smith V M, Bass T A 1982 Communication for the health care team. Harper & Row, London.

United Kingdom Central Council for Nurses Midwives and Health Visitors 1992 Code of professional conduct, 3rd edn. London.

Zander A 1979 The psychology of group processes. Annual review of psychology. 30, 417–452.

The nurse as a reflective practitioner

CONTENTS

7

The nurse as a professional carer

Tepi Corbett

INTRODUCTION

Nursing has undergone many fascinating changes in the past few decades, particularly through the emergence, in the 1970s, of a profess-ional reform movement called 'New Nursing' (Salvage 1992). A central element in the ideology of New Nursing was the relationship between the nurse and the patient. The focus of care moved away from a medical, disease-orientated approach to a person-centred, individualised model. Here the patient was seen as an active participant in, rather than a passive recipient of care. In the same context, the caring role of the nurse no longer centred on the biological functions of the patient but extended to the psycho-social aspects of the individual.

The movement not only addressed the nature of interaction between the patient and the nurse but also the nurse's status and authority. The stereotype of the nurse as a handmaiden to the doctor was being challenged. The quest for equality and autonomy amongst nurses became heightened as nursing theory and models of nursing became established.

Nurses began to see themselves as practitioners in their own right, having and accepting responsibility for making decisions about nursing practice. The nurse/patient relationship was identified as a mark of professional nursing.

Salvage's exploration of New Nursing, carried out from a committed, yet critical nursing perspective, affirms the viewpoint of Gilling (1992), who said '. . . . nursing can confidently call itself a profession, although in certain areas it is only just fulfilling this role' (Gilling 1992).

Table 7.1 Criteria of professionalism attributed to nursing—adapted from Gilling 1992

Criteria of Professionalism	In Nursing
Body of knowledge	Initially derived from medical knowledge; now growing in defining nursing interventions models.
Regulating council	Standards of nursing defined by the United Kingdom Central Council for Nursing, Midwifery and Health Visiting (UKCC).
Client benefit	Patients trust and are confident in the ability of the nurse to perform to a particular standard in meeting their care needs.
Code of conduct	Regulation of the profession through the Professional Code of Conduct (UKCC 1992).
Advancement of knowledge	Continuing post-registration education of nurses—The Future of Professional Practice (UKCC 1994).
Autonomy and equality	Becoming more autonomous: Scope of Professional Practice (UKCC 1992).

Without entering into debate on the professional status of nursing, it is appropriate to reflect on other views of professionalism adapted from that of Gilling's (1992) and outlined in Table 7.1.

In determining a viewpoint of the professional status of nursing the role of the nurse will need to be explored. The evidence shows that caring has consistently formed a highly symbolic component of that role. Concurrently with the nature of nursing, the nature of caring has taken on different dimensions. From the extreme of the disease-orientated procedural and highly mechanistic, impersonal approach, the focus has moved to the recognition of the uniqueness of individuals in the caring situation. Both patient and nurse are now allowed to enter into an intensely interpersonal relationship. The patient is empowered to do so through becoming a better informed participant in the nurse's care; the nurse by the virtue of being a professional carer.

Undertaking personal living activities in sustained intimacy is the privilege of nursing. Caring in this closely interpersonal context, however, is far from easy. It carries a high risk of personal distress and trauma as 'the paradox of nursing is that it can be at one and the same time the spirit of great joy but also of great suffering' (Kirby & Slevin 1992, p.67). It is the expression of that joy and suffering which is shared by patient and nurse through communication. Indeed, meaningful, informed and sensitive interpersonal communication is caring in action.

PUBLIC PERCEPTION OF THE NURSE

The case described in Box 7.1 illustrates one of the extreme images that the public has of a nurse: an administering angel who saves lives as an everyday part of her life and work and does not demand recognition for this service. It implies almost saintly qualities of purity and virtue, whether actual or imagined, within the individual.

Box 7.1 Road accident—a true story

It was a wet and drizzly September morning. The road was busy but traffic was flowing freely as Paul was giving Marie a lift to the hospital where she worked. Suddenly Paul braked hard to avoid an accident which had only just happened. 'You ought to go and see if there is anything that you can do', said Paul, and with that he pulled his car to the roadside just beyond where the accident had happened.

They both got out of the car and hurried to the scene of the accident. A young girl had been knocked off her motor scooter and was lying on the ground. A crowd was forming as people were beginning to gather.

'Let the nurse through, she knows what to do' said Paul. The crowd parted as if pushed aside. Marie bent down and began to attend to the girl who was obviously very badly injured. She appeared unconscious, her leg had been traumatically amputated and blood was pulsating freely from what remained of her leg. In a second, almost as if by intuition, Marie cleared the girl's airway, asked for Paul's tie and used this as a tourniquet round the girl's thigh and stopped the flow of blood.

An ambulance arrived. Marie told the ambulancemen what she had done, left them to carry on with the rest and continued on her way to work.

The headlines in the local newspaper the next day read 'Nameless administering angel saves the life of an accident victim'. A detailed account was given by eyewitnesses of how the nameless nurse had vanished into the crowd without wanting recognition for what she had done.

The image outlined in Box 7.1 coincides with the views held of nurses in the Middle Ages, when some of them were even given the title of saint (Goward 1992). Corresponding viewpoints were found during the Nightingale era when nursing became reinstated as a vocation and service of special value in the eyes of God (Skeet & Nightingale 1980). It embodied the virtues of servility and loyalty in return for little financial reward.

The above image may not be as extreme as it initially appears. Even today some people perceive the nurse as a person who is there to provide the all important human link with living. Henderson (1969) encapsulates this into the nurse being '. . . . the consciousness of the unconscious, the love of life of the suicidal, the leg of the amputee, the eyes of the newly blind, the means of locomotion for the infant, knowledge and confidence for the young mother, a will for those too weak or withdrawn to speak' (Henderson 1969, p.5).

Although nurses are generally held in high esteem, there is a less favourable viewpoint. A popular stereotypical image of nurses is that they have sexually permissive or unconventional attitudes. Female nurses are frequently labelled and depicted as sex symbols. As the adoption of specific uniforms induces certain expectations in the public (Saunders 1986), the portrayal of the nurse's uniform as a short white skirt and black stockings reinforces this image. Male nurses do not escape labelling either. They are frequently assumed to be gay because they have chosen a female oriented profession. These images are, regrettably, reinforced by the media through the well known 'Carry-on' films and television comedy.

Both the positive and negative images described above are ones which are found in the social stereotyping of a nurse. The effect this has is that once a person is recognised as belonging to a particular group of people, she is attributed with the characteristics of that group, irrespective of any individual characteristics (Saunders 1986). This may well influence those young people who are contemplating making nursing their career, particularly if the level of parental support is diminished because of the adverse perceptions of the nurse stereotype. Fortunately there is evidence suggesting the initial effects of stereotyping may only be transient and that 'the follow-up behaviour is a crucial factor in establishing a lasting impression that will endure for the period of interaction' (Saunders 1986) and which will eliminate the effects of stereotyping. Consider Activity 7.1.

Activity 7.1 A personal image of nursing

Using the above text as your starting point draw up a list of attributes related to the image of a nurse that:
- you held before you started your education programme;
- your parents/partner held before you started your education programme.

Reflect on these . . .

How has your professional socialisation affected your viewpoint and that of your parents/partner?

The public perception of a nurse is an issue of some importance. Nurses are key players in a multidisciplinary health care team, promoting and restoring the health in society. Attributing qualities, such as professional competence, frequently occurs before encounters between individuals take place. Therefore the image presented to the public is significant.

If nurses are to influence the way in which the public view them, they need to understand the concepts that determine how person perceptions are formed.

A MODEL OF PERSON PERCEPTION

Self-awareness

The central facet of any social interaction is the way that individuals perceive themselves and those with whom they interact. Perception of self, or self-awareness, is an essential part of the process of becoming a nurse. Nurses are frequently required to reflect on learning experiences so they might benefit from hindsight. Morrison & Burnard (1991) state that 'unless we develop the skill of becoming self-aware, we may well lose the ability to be reflective. The very act of reflecting on who we are helps us to reflect, also, upon what we do . . . . to care for others we must know ourselves'.

The concepts of self-awareness are complex. Ellis (1992) and Morrison & Burnard (1991) conclude that there are a number of dimensions within the outer and inner experience of self which are intimately bound up with our relationships with others.

Perceptions of self and others are highly interdependent processes. People constantly observe those around them and formulate opinions about what they are like and how they might behave. Even in a short space of time impressions can be formed and judgements made about individuals based upon personal factors. Hargie & Marshall (1986) suggest that the gender, age, physical appearance and dress of the individuals determine, to a degree, how they are perceived by others.

Personal factors

Hargie & Marshall (1986) suggest that women are perceived as gentle, warm and tactful whereas men are assertive, rational and unemotional. Women are considered better communicators; they smile more, gaze more directly at others, sit or stand closer to people and read non-verbal cues such as facial expressions, body movements and changes in the tone of voice more accurately. They point out that it still remains true that males and females who deviate markedly from their expected sex role behaviour are likely to encounter problems during social interaction.

Age is an important determinant of social relations and age grading is a significant influence in the structure of some cultures. Calendar age is considered a relevant factor in terms of seniority, level of responsibility, promotion and pay. It may be more difficult for young professionals to gain the confidence of the patient than a mature person. Older people are generally viewed as being more competent in what they do whilst the young are considered 'radical, rebellious and adventurers' (Gahagan 1980). Bromley (1974) also identifies age-related changes in self-awareness, perception of others and the control and expression of feelings.

Physical appearances are also used to make judgements of people. Physically attractive persons are viewed more favourably and are responded to more readily in the first instance. It is only subsequently that other attributes of interpersonal attraction, such as personality, professional approach and interactive style come into the equation.

Clothes are also a part of the perceptual cues to which others respond. They can indicate the occupation and professional status of an individual and figure predominantly in stereotyping. A smart uniform may attract respect and suggest competence in its wearer, whereas an unkempt dress is likely to infer lack of concern and carelessness.

Situational factors

Perceptions of others are not only governed by personal factors but also by situations in which social interactions occur. Each situation, whether it be casual, serious or humorous conveys different impressions. The same person may be perceived totally differently in each situation. This is because individuals adopt diverse roles (see Chapter 3) each of which carry distinct norms that are highly predictive of aspects of behaviour. For example, professional roles carry with them a degree of achieved status which assumes a certain type of behaviour. Some professionals are expected to comply with a code of conduct that lays down guiding principles covering a range of situations. Person perception, then, is an intricate process consisting of three main interrelated components of self-awareness, personal factors and situational factors, see Figure 7.1.

Activity 7.2 Person perception

- Reflect on the occasion when you first met the person in charge of your clinical placement.
What was your first impression?
Has your impression subsequently changed and if so, or indeed if not, what do you think the reason for this to be?
- Identify a person whom you know both in a professional and social context.
How do you view the individual in the different situations?

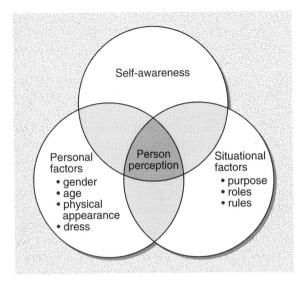

Figure 7.1 Components of person perception

ATTRIBUTION THEORY

It is necessary to differentiate between the perception of an object and the perception of a person. The former is a relatively objective process whereas the latter can be highly subjective.

One person's perception of another is that of a human who shares similar characteristics. Such perceptions are not based solely on the observed characteristics of the person. An attempt is made to attribute causes to why the characteristics are present. Heider (1958) refers to this as attributing causal power to understanding and predicting the behaviour of others. The causes of behaviour may be due to both factors within the person and outwith the person in her physical or social environment (Kelly 1955). It can never be certain whether the behaviour is caused by a psychological characteristic or by social pressures and expectations. During the process of attribution there has to be an awareness of the information held by the observer and the situation in which the behaviour occurs.

The sources that typically affect attribution (Kelly 1955), and which must be taken into account are:

- Distinctiveness.
- Consensus.
- Consistency.

Distinctiveness

Distinctiveness is concerned with the target of behaviour. For example, a father portrays extreme anger towards his son because the son has disobeyed him. Distinctiveness is high when the father's anger is directed only at his son; it is low when his anger is directed towards a large number of people in the room.

In the former situation it may be assumed that the anger is a product of his son's behaviour in their joint situation. In the latter, the father's anger is portrayed in many contexts and could be attributed to his personality as he appears the only common factor in the prevailing situation. Where the factor of distinctiveness is low the causes of behaviour may be more confidently assigned to something within the person (Gahagan 1980).

Consensus

Consensus refers to the degree to which people behave in the same way in a particular situation. Taking the previous example, consensus would be high if everyone who was affected by the disobeyance showed anger towards the son. This indicates that it is the situation that is the cause of behaviour rather than the personality of the individuals. In exploring the concept of person perception, it is low consensus that provides useful information about an individual. For example, if a person acted in a humorous manner during a funeral service, it would indicate a particular characteristic of that individual.

Consistency

The concept of consistency can be described in the example of the disobeying son. If the father's anger only occured on the single occasion, and was never repeated, it could be assumed that the behaviour was a product of the situation. If, however, the father displayed anger repeatedly in similar situations, the assumption would be that the cause of the behaviour is attributed to the person.

It has been shown that even where the context and the behaviour are identical, there can be different causal attributions (Jones & Nisbett 1972). This emphasises that although, through the process of person perception, cause and effect judgements about an individual can be made, alternative explanations cannot be disregarded.

Attribution theory outlines the ways in which observations may be interpreted, but does not provide scientific evidence about the correctness of the attributions. People interpret behaviour differently.

The perception of a person is likely to be dependent on the observer, and is thus variable.

THE NURSE/PATIENT RELATIONSHIP

As determined earlier, since the 1970s there has been a marked shift in the focus of nursing care, and a consequent change in the relationship between the nurse and the patient. Patients have become full partners in their care whereby they, and their significant others, are now empowered to contribute fully to any decision making processes in relation to their own welfare.

The emphasis on health promotion has increased in recent years and, as a result, society as a whole has become much better informed about health related issues. Government initiatives such as Working for Patients (DOH 1989), Caring for People (DOH 1989) and Health of the Nation (DOH 1992) together with much wider and realistic media coverage, have heightened people's awareness of their entitlements, rights and responsibilities. They now question more readily the type and standard of care they experience.

The evolving role of the patient and the changing role of the nurse have affected the relationship between the nurse and the patient. The romantic notion of the nurse mopping the fevered brow no longer exists. Technological advances have meant that nurses increasingly 'care' through the use of machinery which 'allows', or indeed demands, the nurse to distance herself from a close interpersonal relationship with the patient. In addition, as economy driven values increase their hold—marketplace ideology— fewer qualified

nurses are involved in the direct delivery of care. The professionals with greatest experience are involved more in the administration and management of health care services. In the extreme, care delivered by a qualified practitioner may be seen as an unaffordable luxury. This, of course, is unacceptable.

Nursing must not take a retrograde step and fall back into providing routine, task orientated physical care for a patient who will become a passive recipient of that care. Instead, the care must be collaborative, holistic and appropriate to the needs of the patient. In fact, the Code of Professional Conduct (UKCC 1992), designed to safeguard the patient, demands that nurses are accountable, through appropriate conduct, for just that type and quality of nursing care. They must 'recognise and respect the uniqueness and dignity of each patient and client, and respond to their need for care, irrespective of their ethnic origin, religious beliefs, personal attributes, the nature of their health problem or any other factor'.

Despite all the changes that have occurred, one constant element remains; the intimate and unique nature of the relationship between the nurse and the patient.

Factors affecting a quality relationship

To be able to determine the quality of the nurse/patient relationship it is necessary to consider some significant features that such a relationship should contain.

Rogers (1974) suggests that the core components of a helping relationship are warmth and genuineness, empathetic understanding and unconditional positive regard. The elements identified are necessary to secure constructive change for the patient in a therapeutic situation in which caring approaches are adopted. A consideration of additional features such as concreteness, immediacy and confrontation (Carkhuff 1968) would further facilitate a positive outcome.

Burnard (1990), through his exploration of the concepts of warmth and genuineness, argues that these are subjective notions. The perception of personal qualities of another is individual and based on individual experience. People may consider themselves to be 'warm' but this is not necessarily how others see them, perhaps because of cultural differences. Being warm and genuine is not a practical skill but a frame of mind. It is an attitude of acceptance, a respect for the uniqueness of the individual: the nurse for the patient who is in need of care; the patient for the nurse who has a genuine professional interest in promoting the patient's welfare. To achieve warmth and genuineness in a patient/nurse relationship there is no need for profound intimacy between individuals. What is needed is the creation of a climate where the patient feels safe; where there is sharing of insights, opinions and thoughts.

Rogers (1974) identifies this as caring deeply or fully accepting the patient and Authier (1986) as total listening. These are the characteristics of a situation in which the patient, who has come for help, becomes aware that the nurse understands how she feels, accepts her right to make decisions and helps her to develop strategies for positive change.

Empathetic understanding is a special dimension in the building of a caring relationship. It is, in dictionary terms, 'the power of identifying oneself mentally with a person or object of contemplation' (Allen 1990). It is not sympathy for a person's situation or dilemma but an ability to objectively reflect on the feelings of a patient, which she may or may not have expressed in words. It implies acceptance and respect, without prejudice, of the uniqueness of the individual without any inference of agreement or disagreement, approval or disapproval; it is to perceive the world as the patient does. In the words of Scheler (cited in Kirby & Slevin 1992) 'It is indeed a case of feeling the other's feelings, not knowing it, nor judging that the other has it; but it is not the same as going through the experience itself'.

Rogers (1974) warns of the dangers of becoming lost 'in the strange and bizarre world of the other' particularly when dealing with emotionally disturbed people. Here, in an attempt to predict and prevent what could potentially be an unhelpful situation, the importance of being able to reflect must be highlighted. A truly reflective practitioner is one who is able to add to the quality of the caring relationship through empathetic understanding. Not as a counsellor, for this is a distinct activity of a professional trained for the purpose, but using counselling skills (Ellis 1992).

Clause 7 in the Code of Professional Conduct (UKCC 1992) sets out some of the parameters of care for which the nurse is accountable. It describes what Rogers (1974) terms 'unconditional positive regard'. The patient is accepted without condition, without bias. Consider the scenario in Box 7. 2.

The case of a rapist murderer is an example of an occasion when the nurse may have strong preconceived ideas and feelings about the patient. As such, the situation may become emotive. Nurses must focus on their understanding of the factors which influence the processes not only of person perception but also of self perception. This is particularly important in relation to impression formation where emotion may well present a challenge to the quality of the caring relationship. To have unconditional positive regard for a patient implies a notion of goodness in that patient (Burnard 1990). To a nurse, particularly a junior nurse, this may be difficult with the result

---

Box 7.2   Case of a rapist murderer

John, a 26-year-old builder, was found guilty of a brutal rape and murder of a 14-year-old schoolgirl six years ago. He was sentenced to life imprisonment.

John's behaviour throughout his time in prison had been exemplary. He did not communicate with other prisoners; he was what the prison warder called a 'loner'. He was allowed to undertake maintenance duties in the prison which he appeared to enjoy.

Ten days ago John was replacing some roof tiles on a three-storey prison building when he slipped and fell onto the ground sustaining serious head injuries. He was taken to the closest neurosurgery unit rather than to the prison hospital which was not equipped to deal with such a serious case. He was unconscious for a week but was now showing signs of improvement.

Imagine that you are a senior student on the ward and a part of the nursing team caring for John. What are your personal feelings towards John? How do you feel about having to care for him?

that the appropriateness (in terms of quality) of the nurse/patient relationship is diminished. See Activity 7.3.

Activity 7.3

Describe how you would help a new junior nurse on the ward to enter into a quality helping relationship with the patient in the scenario identified in Box 7. 2

The concept of concreteness (Carkhuff 1968) relates to mutual and accurate understanding of the vocabulary that the patient uses, particularly to describe her emotions. Words such as 'sad' and 'happy' are very subjective. The nurse needs to be definite about the meaning of words in the context of the individual patient. The depth of understanding of the other is an important determinant of the quality of the caring relationship.

It is also relevant to consider the immediacy of the feelings that the patient is describing. This refers to the current situation, not to the past or to the future. The focus needs to be on how things are 'today' to promote spontaneous disclosure and open communication and thus enhance the effectiveness of the caring relationship. For example, when the patient refers to her anxiety about the impending results of a recent investigation, it is important to determine how she feels about the investigation right now and not how she felt about it before it took place.

Sometimes people make generalisations about events, people and feelings. In order to help patients, it may be necessary to confront them, not in an aggressive way, but rather to coax them to find out 'the truth'. This may be relevant in a case where an elderly gentleman who has been brought into hospital for a hip replacement and thinks that hospitals are places where people come to die rather than to get better. To increase the patient's motivation to recover, the nurse needs to be able to help him to develop a more positive attitude; a sense of optimism about the outcome and benefits of the operation, through the process of confrontation.

By exploring the essential components of a caring relationship, as proposed by Rogers (1974) and Carkhuff (1968), it becomes clear that the extent to which these are present or absent affects the quality of the caring relationship between a nurse and a patient.

COMMUNICATING IN THE WORK ENVIRONMENT

Communication is fundamental to all professional relationships in the work environment, in what Ellis (1992) calls 'a web of relationships'. The professional needs to be able to discriminate between the different channels and styles of communication and select the most appropriate ones for the prevailing situation.

Groenman et al (1992) differentiate between two directions associated with communication: horizontal and vertical. Horizontal direction refers to an interaction between individuals whose status, either ascribed or assumed, is the same. Their powers of decision making correspond both in terms of level and extent; the individuals are of equal importance or seniority in the hierarchy. Communication here is normally two-way with each individual having equal say as partners.

In vertical communication the flow is generally one way between individuals who have disparate power and/or status. Here, the 'senior' gives orders either in writing or verbally. The 'junior' is not expected to contribute, it is the senior person who makes the decisions for the subordinate. See Activity 7.4.

Activity 7.4   Professional relationships

Identify the professional relationships that you have encountered during your education programme. Consider each one in turn and categorise these in terms of their direction.
Repeat the activity in relation to your personal relationships.

In Activity 7.4 there may be difficulty in discerning which of the polarities applied to each situation. This is not surprising as the majority would be sited between the two extremes, and be of mixed direction.

Reflecting upon the changing roles of a doctor and a nurse, and a nurse and a patient, it would seem that, over time, the direction has changed from the vertical pole towards the horizontal pole as the formality versus informality of the relationship has altered.

Communication style and tone may require adjustment, depending on the direction of the communication. This highlights the fact that the professional must be able to discern and discriminate between the roles of the sender and the receiver, and the nature of the message.

ENVIRONMENTAL INFLUENCES ON COMMUNICATION

Communication may become ineffective when any of the fundamental components—the sender, message, receiver or context—is inappropriate or faulty. Communication is seldom faultless.

Having explored some of the dimensions of social influence on self and person perception, and determined the real significance of first impressions it is necessary to recognise them as forces in the context in which interaction occurs i.e. the physical environment.

When buying property, the purchaser will have experienced the concept of the 'ambience' of the houses viewed. The smells, sights and even sounds of a place may have strongly influenced opinion in relation to whether the property was suitable. In fact, the property press, in its advice to vendors, suggests that the smell of such things as fresh ground coffee, newly baked bread and cakes may influence potential buyers favourably. Strong smells of spicy foods and stale vegetables could have an adverse effect. When visiting the doctor's or dentist's surgery, the person's confidence in the quality of service offered may well be influenced by first impressions of the waiting room. A calm and relaxed atmosphere will create confidence and reduce anxiety.

Most new hospitals, hospices and private clinics now have comfortable reception areas usually staffed by trained receptionists who will endeavour to allay the anxieties of clients and relatives. Hargie et al (1981) refer to this as 'the provision of creature comforts' designed to make individuals welcome and induce confidence in a situation that can be very stressful. The wider use of muted colours which are 'pleasing to the eye', appropriate lighting, colourful soft furnishings, pictures on the walls and soothing music all function as distractions in situations which might provoke strong emotions. Unfortunately there still exist a number of old hospitals and clinics where the starkness, unattractive colour schemes and strong smells of disinfectants add to the fears of patients and visitors. See Activity 7.5.

***

Activity 7.5 The effects of the physical environment on communication

Reflect on occasions when you have attended an interview:
- at school/college to see the headteacher or form teacher;
- for a job/entry to your current education programme;
- with your personal tutor/academic supervisor.

What was the physical setting of the environment like? How did it affect you?

***

The physical layout of the room in which meetings or group work take place is a powerful determinant in the kind and quality of interaction that takes place (McMaster 1986). The tone of the meeting is frequently influenced by such factors as the type and arrangement of seating. This is an important factor to keep in mind when preparing an environment where interaction will take place. It is said that hostility, dispute or confrontation are found to occur more frequently in face-to-face or head-on situations whereas cooperation, friendliness and acceptance are enhanced by seating which is side-by-side. In each of the situations, a strong contributory factor will be the distance i. e. the proximity between individuals. Generally the shorter the distance, the more friendly the encounter. It is important to consider variations which result from cultural differences. For example, amongst Arabs, closer physical proximity, face-to-face interaction and eye contact is expected in all situations. In fact, culture and communication is of great significance, particularly for those professionals who function in multi-cultural societies. Unless nurses can appreciate these cultural differences they may be faced with awkward situations which could lead to serious misunderstandings. Brislin (1981) provides an important text in this area.

THE INFLUENCE OF STRESS ON COMMUNICATION

Stress is a common phenomenon within the health care professions. In scientific terms Snowley (1992) defines stress as 'any change within a system induced by an external force'. The external forces are manifold, but with health care professionals stress is most commonly the result of emotional tensions associated with the nature of their work. The immense and constant emotional commitment required of nurses in difficult caring situations may manifest in stress, for example when nurses do not appear to be able to help the patient in a life-threatening situation. The effects of stress are potentially harmful and for this reason the importance and methods of managing stress have, in the recent years, received a good deal of attention. It is not the intention of this text to explore these methods in any depth here. Authors to whom the reader is directed include Bailey & Clarke (1989), Bond (1986), and Sutherland & Cooper (1990) all of who treat the subject admirably in the context of caring and health care professionals. The purpose of this text is merely to site stress in the context of communication (see Activity 7.6).

Activity 7.6 The effects of stress on communication

- Identify three instances in your personal life that you have found particularly stressful.
- List the most stressful events that you have experienced associated with your studies.
How did you feel psychologically and how did it affect you physically?
Compare your views with your group members in an attempt to determine what caused the instances to be stressful.

In working through Activity 7.6, one of the stressful events that may be identified is attending a competitive interview for a job or a place on a course. If the event is crucial, whereby one's future depends on it, the more likely that stress response symptoms will be experienced. Pounding of the heart, dryness of the mouth, nervous twitching or fidgeting, frequent urination, sweating of the palms, and forgetting the things that had been read in preparation for the event, are typical.

Should the event prove to be better than expected then the stress responses may well be minimal. However, if previous experiences have been unpleasant, responses will be heightened (Bailey & Clarke 1989).

The significance of the above is that stress may well influence communication and as such may lead to the misinterpretation of an individual's behaviour. The level of eye contact may be decreased which may be an indication of lack of attention or submissiveness. The spatial needs of the person experiencing stress will probably be altered as physical closeness may well interfere with the security needs of the person, the closer the 'intruder' the more vulnerable the person feels. Nurses may have experienced the situation of being cornered, which increases stress still further. Physical and psychological distances play an important role in the communication process, particularly in terms of self-disclosure in the caring relationship.

Nurses must, however, remember that there is a great deal of diversity between different cultures. For example in a number of oriental cultures the appropriateness of interaction distance is determined by status. Because of the cultural teachings of humility, modesty and subordination, too close a proximity would indicate insubordination. Similarly, people from Asian cultures indicate respect by allowing more space, keeping their heads low and averting their eyes. The Americans, in turn, would view this sort of passive behaviour as indicative of an individual who is distant, submissive or evasive. Although the above are generalisations, they signify the importance of being aware of cultural variations in order to prevent misinterpretation of behaviour manifested by stress.

Individuals experiencing stress are likely to show behaviour which is totally atypical for them. For example, a person may become verbally very aggressive and/or abusive. This may produce strong emotions in others who are involved and make the situation a very complex one to handle. This type of situation is a common occurrence in an Accident and Emergency department, although in a great number of instances the aggression is due to intoxication by either drugs or alcohol.

Managing information

Hospitalisation in itself induces stress, most commonly caused by ineffective communication. Patients and their significant others may be given information in a format that they do not understand (jargon). They are not able to be assertive enough to ask for an explanation with the result that their stress is increased due to lack of understanding. Stress also affects the individual's ability to concentrate; the attention span may be greatly reduced leading to a lack of ability to recall information (Newell 1994). This means that if information is given in a quantity too great for an individual to manage then information overload and forgetfulness will occur. It does not matter whether the news is good or bad, the patients and their significant others just do not remember what they have been told. Alternatively they may focus on words like cancer, heart attack and pain out of context of the explanation which accompanied these (Davis 1984); issues may have been magnified out of all proportion. There may be incongruence between understanding and, for example, non-verbal communication portrayed by the patients. An affirmatory nodding of the head may occur, which generally would indicate that the information has been understood. In this context, however, it would be erroneous to think so.

The moral of the above is that any stress, either overt or indeed covert, must be dealt with appropriately to enhance optimum communication between individuals in an interactive situation, either in a caring relationship or work situation.

LANGUAGE CODES AND PROFESSIONAL JARGON

Social functions of language between the professionals include the sharing of verbal signs and jargon within that 'speech community'. This acts as a link between the individuals; it is a public sign of 'belonging' to a professional group. As one of the first activities within a profession, a new recruit will endeavour to learn the language that is common to the members of that group.

Language differences which result from the use of jargon and technical terms between the patient and the carer may interfere with communication. The basic necessity of communication is to understand the utterances of others and if jargon is used a gap in comprehension may occur. Some words may also have frightening connotations for the patient. For example the use of the word 'pneumonia' to some, and particularly to elderly people, may imply a critical life-threatening situation. They are not aware of the difference in prognosis which has resulted from the use of antibiotic or, more recently, antiviral drugs. This lack of comprehension will precipitate stress and result in even greater communication problems as we have seen above.

There are language differences between people from different social backgrounds which would indicate the type of language code, restricted or elaborated, that needs to to be used to ensure understanding. It is appropriate to highlight the fact that when people become ill, hospitalised or dependent on a carer their ability to understand may be altered. There is often an assumption that a nurse or a doctor will fully understand what is happening to patients or what is expected of them in their sick role and, because of this, patients are not given sufficient explanation. This will lead to additional anxiety and stress which may present in further communication problems.

It becomes abundantly clear that the style of language chosen, either literary or vernacular, is contextualised not only by the topic of conversation but also by the setting and the relationship between the people involved.

COMMUNICATING WITH DIFFERENT CLIENT GROUPS

The pivotal component of any interpersonal relationship is communication, not least of all in the professional relationship between the nurse, the patient and the patient's family and friends. A large part of that relationship involves face-to-face interaction and professionals are expected to have appropriate knowledge of, and expertise in, communication skills. Hargie (1986) refers to these as social skills which are 'a set of goal orientated, inter-related, situationally appropriate social behaviours which can be learnt and which are under the control of the individual'.

Most individuals are perfectly capable of using social skills in everyday lives as private citizens. However, it is not uncommon for new entrants to the profession to exclaim, prior to their first visit to the clinical areas, 'what do I say to them; how do I talk to them?' A person not normally perturbed about talking to someone can find this situation difficult. It is no longer a strictly 'social' one where the individuals engage in informal conversation but rather a professional caring situation where the roles being enacted are those of a carer and a person needing care. The role of the carer conjectures certain types of behaviour, attitudes and values. The carer is expected to be concerned about the well-being of the patient; to portray a non-judgemental approach to the patient's behaviour regardless of her own values and beliefs and to deal effectively with those who exhibit anti-social behaviour. The carer must be able to distance herself from her own personal needs.

For the relationship between the nurse and the patient to be a quality helping relationship, it needs to contain elements such as empathy, warmth and understanding and unconditional positive regard. These qualities will be portrayed through attending, listening and responding.

Paying attention to a patient in any caring situation is a positive way in which to convey warmth. Burnard (1991) refers to this as staying awake 'to be fully present in the moment that is being lived'. It involves being physically and psychologically with the patient. It is demonstrated mainly through non-verbal behaviour, for example, maintaining eye contact but not staring; leaning forward but respecting the spatial needs of the patient to convey interest; nodding as a confirmation of interest to what the patient is saying. Cognisance of cultural influences, factors which influence person perception and the context of the interaction are of paramount importance. The patient must be viewed within her frame of reference with empathetic understanding.

Non-verbal communication is also a significant component of listening. A person involved in an exchange of opinions with a friend may exclaim: 'You are not listening to what I am saying!' The intentional words, phrases and sentences may well have been heard but what has gone unnoticed

are the appearances, mannerisms and the context of the interaction. The interpretation of the meaning of the communication thus becomes flawed. Listening, therefore, is an active process which demands the listener to concentrate on the multi-sensory cues, in search for the meaning and understanding portrayed by the speaker. Smith (1986) proposes that people listen to acquire information; to empathise; to discriminate between a variety of moods of the speaker; to evaluate alternatives in choosing an appropriate course of action; to appreciate beauty, order and symmetry. Effective listening will, therefore, enhance self-control, diminish misunderstanding and frustration and generally enhance the quality of interpersonal relationships.

Attending and listening are not only concerned with non-verbal behaviour; they are also about portraying receptiveness and understanding through encouraging the patient to express feelings and ideas in a supportive but not in a defensive way. The carer will seek to help the patient to convey meaning through verbal signals which indicate interest in what the patient wishes to express by using a rhetorical question; 'is that so' or 'tell me about it'. In all of this, the patient directs the flow of conversation and the carer prompts her to explore issues further.

Responding effectively to patients in caring situations amounts to verbal and non-verbal behaviours being portrayed in such a way as to reflect sensitivity, compassion and professional concern (see Box 7.3).

Box 7.3 Sensitive, compassionate and concerned communication

- *Sensitivity* is evidenced through the recognition of the uniqueness of the individuals, the way in which they perceive the world around them and the social, cultural and emotional context of their feelings.
- *Compassion* embodies forgetting oneself, suspending judgement and entering the world of the patient on her terms.
- *Professional concern* encompasses the collaborative exploration of the problems of the patient with unconditional positive regard, establishment of mutual understanding and common goals and agreeing interventions directed towards the achievement of optimum well-being.

There is strong evidence to suggest that professionals need to learn the skills which are essential for the establishment and maintenance of a quality caring relationship with clients and patients. Burnard (1990), Burnard & Morrison (1991), Davis (1984), and Newell (1994) all address this issue in depth.

By recognising the concept of 'situationally appropriate' the nurse needs to consider both the social context and the frame of reference of the different client groups with whom health care professionals interact. Although the basic principles of effective communication apply, there are three distinct components which demand special emphasis: children, adults and people with learning disabilities.

Communicating with children

Caring for children is a very specialist area of professional practice, particularly in an era in which the rights of children have been made explicit (Children Act 1989 and Department of Health 1991). The professionals can provide appropriate care to the sick child only if they are familiar with the normal developmental stages that children undergo to achieve physical and intellectual potential.

Children are not small versions of adults, nor are they carbon copies of their parents, but individuals within their own right with the capacity to become unique adults. Their prime task, on arrival into the world, is to discover themselves and their immediate environment of which they are acutely aware. It is through communication that children form relationships not only with other humans but also with the social world around them.

Effective communication is never easy but communicating with children requires a special and different approach. Although the basic components are the same, particular emphasis needs to be placed on thorough appreciation of the developing abilities and understanding of children. The professional needs to adopt different techniques that take account of the stage of language development and communication skill of the child.

The use of appropriate communication approaches between the sick child and the professional enhances the development of the caring relationship in which the child is permitted not only to express her needs but also to have those needs met. Barlow (1992) enforces this by stating that 'the paediatric nurse requires heightened skills in observation which, when combined with professional knowledge, will enable her to interpret a child's behaviour, body language and physical symptoms . . . non-verbal communication is particularly important where the child is unable to express her needs and feelings in words' (Barlow 1992).

Non-verbal signals of thoughts and feelings are constantly displayed by individuals. The way an adult interacts with a child by smiling, frowning, cuddling and the use of gestures all communicate the extent of caring. This is particularly important as non-verbal communication has great meaning to children before they understand words. Getting down to the child's level, both mentally and physically, using gentle speech and movement enhances the child's trust and security.

Adults and children do not react or respond in the same way. A helping professional acknowledges the child's feelings and conveys to her that it is all right to feel happy or sad, pleased or angry. These feelings, however must be channelled into something constructive, for example age-appropriate play activity or, with the older child, talking through the emotions. Play is a pervasive and characteristic part of the behaviour of a normal healthy child through which learning and communication takes place. Children frequently express their feelings and attitudes through drawing and a great deal can be learnt of the child's self image or perception of her parents from the portraits that she draws (Davis 1984).

For communication to be effective, it is also important to discern the language that is familiar to the child. This is not just concerned with intellectual ability but also with the child's own version of words. As children's language frequently mirrors that of their significant others, cognisance of any dialectical and cultural variations is significant. The professional will then be able to ensure that an appropriate linguistic approach is adopted.

Communicating with adults

Meaningless reassurances and generalisations, such as 'you don't have anything to worry about', and 'I know exactly how you are feeling', undermine the intelligence of adult patients. The individual is used to certain social behaviour and routines, the consequences of which she is able to predict. This creates a sense of security and gives order to daily living. Becoming ill, and particularly being admitted to hospital, causes disequilibrium and can become a very threatening experience. It is the professional's responsibility to ensure that this is minimised by providing full explanations about such things as treatment schedules and routines and the reasons for them. Instances such as checking the nameband of a patient the nurse knows, can create great anxiety for some patients. This procedure, although in accordance with regulations, may imply an impersonal, non-entity approach unless explained to the patient.

Hospitalised adults may feel vulnerable, insecure and inadequate being surrounded by authoritative figures. Their independent state has been altered to one in which others decide when they eat and when they go to bed. Even going to the bathroom may involve having to have permission to do so. This may be a threatening experience, where the adult feels powerless and anxious, and may manifest in anger and aggression. Alternatively, the individual may speak more slowly (because of tense vocal cords) and in a higher pitch. The normally articulate adult may make more speech errors and become less coherent (Davis 1984), and her understanding of issues related to her care may well become 'blurred'. All these factors may significantly influence the carer's perception of the person unless she is fully aware of why they might exist.

The effects of role change may be particularly strong when the individual has held, or currently holds a responsible position in her private or work situation. The adult has the right to considerate, socially contextual and respectful care. Addressing individuals as 'pops' or 'sweetie' is inconsiderate and may well be a barrier to a collaborative caring relationship.

Verbal and non-verbal communication supplement, and indeed complement each other. As with children non-verbal behaviour among adults is equally important. Facial expression, body movement and tone of voice give cues about the emotional state of the adult. It must, however, be emphasised that adults do have control over these; they may well be able to conceal their emotions. Similarly, adults are far more conscious of social norms and pressures, such as the prohibition of emotional expression, particularly crying, in males.

Young adults are usually very concerned about their body image and physical appearance. Carers must be aware and respect the individual's feelings about this. Specially sensitive communication, both verbal and non-verbal, is required from those professionals who work with patients who have experienced mutilating interventions, for example, people who have had a stoma or the removal of a breast, and equally patients who have undergone a hysterectomy or a prostatectomy where no physically outward signs are necessarily evident.

It is through the adoption of appropriate patient-contextual communication by the professionals that adult patients are able to move beyond bio-psycho-social immobility to achieve acceptance of their illness and control over their being. They will thus become self-accepting which is a pre-requisite for harmonious inner life.

Communicating with people with learning difficulties

Communication is a fundamental component of each individual's life. Without it a meaningful role in society would not be possible. There are, however, individuals in society who throughout their whole lifespan present with a varying degree of intellectual impairment which affects their bio-psycho-social functioning; these are people who have learning difficulties. Caring for these people is a specialist function which requires professional education in an evolving context of care provision which is now becoming integrated into the general community rather than remaining in the hospital setting.

Each one of these individuals has the need to communicate despite the fact that they may well not be able to understand or use linguistic forms of communication. The emphasis must be on using appropriate approaches of non-verbal communication, yet with the knowledge that some individuals may also have physical incapacities. As in all caring situations the approach must be centred on the specific needs of the individual person.

Because verbal communication may be inappropriate, the nurse must ensure that non-verbal communication becomes deliberate for it to be truly meaningful for people with a learning disability. Distinction must be made between verbal communication and language, for people with a learning disability may well be able to vocalise in a communicative way (Burford 1993).

This chapter has examined channels of expressing non-verbal communication such as facial expression, eye contact, touch, posture and spatial proximity, including some cultural differences related to these. The actions that are involved are normally precisely coordinated and are synchronised with language. People with learning disabilities may not have the ability to do this, a fact which may seriously diminish the meaningfulness of the communication.

It may be an extremely long process that requires immense patience to establish communication with people with learning disabilities. The main difficulty could be the fact that the communication is often one-sided. Most people, whilst leaving a message on an answering machine, will have experienced considerable difficulty and frustration in speaking to a passive recipient. The important factor to remember in relation to communicating with people with learning disabilities is that even the slightest response is encouraging. There is no need to have equal input from each person involved in communication. The person may well be responding equally intensely within her limitations. 'The communication is not about facts or events, rather it is a way of acknowledging each other, sharing feelings and enjoying each other's company' (Burford 1993 p. 286).

To fulfil the main aim of communication in terms of creating and developing a caring relationship, it is wise not to intervene too quickly when inviting a response. Haste may result in misunderstanding which, in turn, may lead to a delay of trust between individuals.

Extreme adaptability on behalf of the professional is required as each individual with a learning disability has different ability. They do not have cultural variations in terms of non-verbal communication, but very individual preferences. Some have acute dislike for close proximity and become very anxious and withdrawn. The essential component of warmth is therefore very difficult to demonstrate for such people. The carer must, therefore, approach each individual in a manner which is acceptable to that individual. Nothing should be done to the person; everything should be done with the person.

CONCLUSION

It is not possible to establish communication with everybody, no matter how hard the carer tries. However, the provision of empathetic understanding, warmth and genuineness and unconditional positive regard towards an individual can be learnt through becoming aware of all the channels through which these can be portrayed.

REFERENCES

Allen R E (ed) 1990 The concise Oxford dictionary of current English 8th edn. Clarendon Press, London.

Authier J 1986 Showing warmth and empathy. In: Hargie O (ed) A handbook of communication skills. Routledge, London, ch. 18.

Bailey R, Clarke M 1989 Stress and coping in nursing. Chapman & Hall, Suffolk.

Barlow S 1992 Children. In: Kenworthy N, Snowley G, Gilling C (eds) Common foundation studies in nursing. Churchill Livingstone, Edinburgh, ch. 14.

Bond M 1986 Stress and self-awareness: a guide for nurses. Heinemann Nursing, Oxford.

Brislin R W 1981 Cross-cultural encounters: face-to-face interaction. Pergammon Press Ltd., Oxford.

Bromley D B 1974 The foundations of social behaviour. In: Radford J, Govier E (eds) A textbook of psychology. Sheldon Press, London, ch. 25.

Buckenham J E, McGrath G 1983 The social reality of nursing. Adis Health Science Press, Australia, ch. 2.

Burford B 1993 Learning disabilities: a handbook of care 2nd edn. Churchill Livingstone, Edinburgh, ch. 12.

Burnard P 1990 Learning human skills: an experiential guide for nurses, 2nd edn. Butterworth-Heinemann Ltd., Oxford.

Carkhuff R R 1968 Helping and human relations. Holt, Rhinehart & Winston, New York.

Davis A J 1984 Listening and responding. C V Mosby Co., Missouri.

Department of Health 1989a Working for patients. HMSO, London.

Department of Health 1989b Caring for people. HMSO, London.

Department of Health 1991 Patient's charter. HMSO, London.

Department of Health 1991 Welfare of children and young people in hospital. HMSO, London.

Department of Health 1992 Health of the nation. HMSO, London.

Ellis R B 1992 The nurse as a communicator. In: Kenworthy N, Snowley G, Gilling C (eds) Common foundation studies in nursing. Churchill Livingstone, Edinburgh, ch. 14.

Gahagan J 1980 The foundations of social behaviour. In: Radford J, Govier E (eds) A textbook of psychology. Sheldon Press, London, ch. 25.

Gilling C 1993 The professional role of the nurse. In: Kenworthy N, Snowley G, Gilling C (eds) Common foundation studies in nursing. Churchill Livingstone, Edinburgh, ch. 14.

Goward P 1992 The development of the nursing profession. In: Kenworthy N, Snowley G, Gilling C (eds) Common foundation studies in nursing. Churchill Livingstone, Edinburgh, ch. 14.

Groenman N H, Slevin O D'A, Buckenham M A 1992 Social and behavioural sciences for nurses. Campion Press Ltd., Edinburgh, Module 5.

Gruending D L 1985 Nursing theory: a vehicle of professionalisation. Journal of Advanced Nursing 10, 6, 553–558.

Hargie O, Marshall P 1986 Interpersonal communication: a theoretical framework. In: Hargie O (ed) A handbook of communication skills. Routledge, London, ch. 2.

Hargie O, Saunders C, Dickson D 1981 Social skills in interpersonal communication. Croom Helm, London.

Heider F 1958 The psychology of interpersonal relations. Wiley, New York.

Henderson V 1969 Basic principles of nursing care. International Council of Nurses, Geneva, revised edition.

Jones E E, Nisbett R E 1972 The actor and the observer: divergent perceptions of the causes of behaviour. In: Jones E E et al (eds) Attribution: perceiving the causes of behaviour. Genevore Learning Group, New Jersey.

Kelly A, 1955 The psychology of personal construct. Norton, New York.

Kirby C, Slevin O 1992 A new curriculum for care. In: Slevin O, Buckenham M (eds) Project 2000. The teachers speak. Innovations in the nursing curriculum. Campion Press Ltd., Edinburgh, ch. 4.

McMaster J 1986 Case conference presentation. In: Hargie O (ed) A handbook of communication skills. Routledge, London, ch. 14.

Morrison P, Burnard P 1991 Caring and communicating: the interpersonal relationship in nursing. Macmillan Education Ltd., London.

Newell R 1994 Interviewing skills for nurses and other health care professionals. A structured approach. Routledge, London.

Rogers C R 1974 On becoming a person, 4th edn. Constable, London.

Salvage J 1992 The new nursing: empowering patients or empowering nurses? In: Robinson J, Gray A, Elkan R (eds) Policy issues in nursing. Open University Press, Milton Keynes, ch. 1.

Saunders C 1986 Opening and closing. In: Hargie O (ed) A handbook of communication skills. Routledge, London, ch. 7.

Skeet M, Nightingale F 1980 Notes on nursing—what it is and what it is not. Churchill Livingstone, Edinburgh.

Smith V 1986 Listening. In: Hargie O (ed) A handbook of communication skills. Routledge, London, ch. 10.

Snowley G 1992 Stress, pain and the individual. In: Kenworthy N, Snowley G, Gilling C Common foundation studies in nursing. Churchill Livingstone, Edinburgh, ch. 4.

Sutherland V J, Cooper C L 1990 Understanding stress. Chapman and Hall, Suffolk.

United Kingdom Central Council for Nursing, Midwifery and Health Visiting 1992 Code of professional conduct 3rd edn. UKCC, London.

United Kingdom Central Council for Nursing, Midwifery and Health Visiting 1992 Scope of professional practice. June. UKCC, London.

United Kingdom Central Council for Nursing, Midwifery and Health Visiting 1994 The Future of Professional Practice, March. UKCC, London.

FURTHER READING

Brislin R W 1981 Cross-cultural encounters. Face-to-face interaction. Pergammon Press Ltd., Oxford. An extensive source of intricacy-associated aspects contributing to cultural differences, their interpretation and approaches for overcoming these, mainly from a psychological perspective.

Burnard P 1990 Learning human skills, 2nd edn. Butterworth Heinemann Ltd., Oxford. A text which shows how nurses can enhance their interpersonal skills and develop counselling and group skills. It provides useful exercises for the individual's self-development.

Hargie O, Marshall P 1986 Interpersonal communication: a theoretical framework. In: Hargie O (ed) A handbook of communication skills. Routledge, London. An excellent text providing a useful theory background to communication.

Home E (ed) 1992 Effective communication, 2nd edn. Wolfe Publishing. Provides examples of difficult situations which require nurses to learn and adopt special communication skills—compilation of articles from the journal Professional Nurse.

Jolley J 1981 The other side of paediatrics. Macmillan Press. A very easy to read text which explores non-medical needs of sick children.

Melia K 1987 Learning and working: the occupational socialisation of nurses. Tavistock, London.

Moloney M 1986 Professionalisation of nursing: current issues and trends. Lippincott, Philadelphia.

Newell R 1994 Interviewing skills for nurses and other health care professionals. A structured approach. Routledge, London. A text which concentrates on the kinds of skills nurses will need to acquire and develop in order to offer the highest quality of care. Provides a number of practical exercises.

Porrit L 1984 Communication: choices for nurses. Longman.

Tschudin V 1991 Counselling skills for nurses 3rd edn. Bailliere Tindall.

8

The mentoring relationship

Patricia East

INTRODUCTION

The advent of Project 2000, with its common foundation programme and establishment of a qualification with greater academic currency for the newly accredited nurse, makes explicit what was implicit in the past: that entrants to nursing are adult learners. If the nurse needs to be successful as a reflective practitioner in both general and specific areas then the learning environment must match this need.

The curriculum framework for communicating and developing in-depth knowledge of the subject matter and skills required must also be linked to the practice of nursing. The use of mentoring programmes has been widely advocated as a means of providing a developmental bridge between theory and practice for the inexperienced nurse entrant. This chapter examines the conceptual bases for mentoring and its application in organisational, educational and nursing settings.

THE ORIGINAL MENTOR

The Greek poet, Homer, tells the story of Odysseus, King of Ithaca, who, whilst away fighting in the Trojan War, entrusted his young son, Telemachus, to the care of a guardian named Mentor. Odysseus was prevented from returning home for 10 years and the goddess Athena, moved by his plight, assumed the appearance of Mentor to make an earthly visit to stir Telemachus into mounting a rescue operation for his father. Thereafter, Athena would appear in the guise of Mentor whenever she wanted to offer support and guidance.

Athena was the daughter of Zeus and had inherited many of her father's powers and qualities, although she was neither all powerful nor all wise. Often connected with war, Athena was also patroness of arts and crafts, occasionally the goddess of medicine and ultimately the goddess of wisdom. Thus Athena combined her practical skills with insight and wisdom and a capacity to work on behalf of others.

Modern ideas about mentoring can therefore be seen to have their roots in mythology. Athena could embody both male and female qualities; her purpose was to support and guide others—be they individuals or the state of Athens—to strive for and to achieve the highest goals. In order to do this Athena took the roles of teacher, adviser, counsellor, sponsor and guide, whenever her support was required. She was also able to integrate the needs of the individual into the wider context. This chapter demonstrates how these are all essential qualities for the role of mentor (see Fig. 8.1).

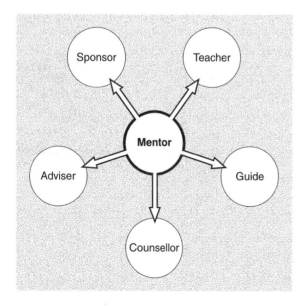

Figure 8.1 The role of the mentor

DEFINING THE ROLE OF MENTOR

While it may not be possible to call on a goddess to act as mentor, some definitions of the role are rooted in this classical ideal. Rowntree's (1981) definition of a mentor as a 'trusted and friendly adviser or guide, especially of someone new to a particular role' is drawn from this origin. In this classical definition the mentor becomes involved in a powerful interpersonal relationship with a less experienced, normally younger person. The relationship involves the engagement of mentor and mentee in the objective and subjective world of each other.

Daloz' (1986) description of a mentor also has classical origins reflected in a Jungian archetypal figure. The mentor represents knowledge, reflection, insight, understanding, good advice, determination and planning; qualities which cannot be mastered alone. Using the metaphor of a journey, Daloz' concern is that the mentor acts as a travelling companion who is more a trusted guide than a tour director.

Daloz refers to the poet Virgil as a classical mentor when he accompanies Dante on his journey through the underworld. This 'mentor supreme' protects, urges forward, explains mysteries, points the way, leaves Dante alone when necessary, translates codes, calms marauding beasts, clears obstacles and encourages—always encourages—helping Dante to find in himself the courage to go on. Embedded in this metaphor is a model for the mentoring role in nurse education. The mentor engenders trust, issues challenges, offers vision, and alternatively supports and challenges the mentee (see Table 8.1).

Virgil knew when to leave Dante, just as mentors eventually need to let go of their mentees. This final point may be linked with Winnicott's (1982) ideas of 'good-enough mothering' and the 'holding environment'. Central to these ideas is the notion that once a child gains a sense of his continuing existence then he is able to successfully separate, initially from his primary caretaker and consequently from others throughout life, without too much anxiety. Kegan (1982) has developed and extended Winnicott's insights across the whole of

Table 8.1 Dante, Virgil and the nurse mentor

VIRGIL	NURSE MENTOR
A well respected authority	A well respected authority
A model poet	A model nurse practitioner
	Appears at the outset to offer support, allay fears of isolation, ignorance and ridicule
Virgil has made this journey before	Nurse mentor has completed her own training and kept up to date with recent developments
	Can act as a guide
Virgil knows the danger spots and can alert Dante in advance—Dante must negotiate the dangers, the pits, the chasms of despair, the cauldrons of boiling blood himself	Nurse mentor knows what lies ahead and can alert her mentee in advance to prepare for the unknown, offer her support and encouragement, challenge and confront when necessary
	Can give advance notice and an overview of the whole process, offer support, facilitate learning, give feedback, constructive criticism and praise
Virgil can understand and speak the languages of the underworld and explain the rules, rituals and symbols to Dante	Nurse mentor understands and can speak in UKCC code and interpret medical terms, academic jargon and the esoteric demands of tutors
	Can translate and de-mystify course requirements
Virgil explains Dante's quest to the damned	Nurse mentor acts on mentee's behalf
	Acts as an advocate
Virgil leaves Dante at the end of his journey	Nurse Mentor recognises mentee's competence
	Allows independence and can separate

life-span developmental psychology, describing a procession of 'holding environments' or 'cultures'. Good mentors ensure that their mentees can recognise that authority has its uses but is limited and that the task of becoming independent involves separation from authority figures and taking on one's own authority.

An important introduction to the concept of mentoring can be found in the work of Levinson et al (1978), which examines the contribution of the mentoring relationship over four phases of adult life. According to Levinson, a mentor is neither a parent nor a peer but a transitional

figure, usually 8–15 years older than the mentee. If the age difference is greater than 20 years the mentor is likely to act in a paternalistic manner; if less than eight years then it is more likely that an intimate, or collaborative peer friendship would ensue in which mentoring would tend to be minimal. In Levinson's definition the mentor facilitates life transitions between the ages of 20 and 40 by allowing the mentee to be a 'novice or apprentice to a more advanced, expert and authoritative adult'. Mentors exemplify the qualities that the mentees wish to attain and their values, virtues and accomplishments are eventually internalised by the mentees. Levinson's work has been criticised on several grounds though primarily for the following reasons:

- Gender bias—the case studies were all male.
- Although Levinson identified the need for a mentor as being common to all men, he did not specify how many of his subjects had mentors which means that a valid evaluation of the role is not possible from his work.
- Levinson's suggestion that mentors are characteristically 8–15 years older than their mentees has been criticised on the grounds that it might be more appropriate to consider the quality and experience of the mentor rather than this arbitrary age criterion.

Despite this criticism, however, Levinson's vivid and detailed description of the mentoring relationship has helped to stimulate the imagination of others.

Early thinking about mentoring drew heavily on the special mythical qualities of the relationship. The claimed advantages of mentoring led to high expectations of the process which in turn led to developments in training and education programmes intended to incorporate these advantages.

These developments were in line with Clutterbuck's (1985) view that the origins of mentoring are to be found in the concept of apprenticeship. In this sense a mentor becomes involved in a relationship which is initiated, sometimes formally, by an organisation in order to achieve results similar to those of the classical relationship, as part of a structured staff develop-

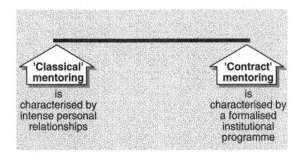

Figure 8.2   The mentoring continuum

ment programme. Managers of staff development programmes began to analyse the functions of the classical relationship so that these could be incorporated into structured training. This led to an emphasis on mentoring as a skills hierarchy with, in some cases, an emphasis on specific outcomes.

The distinction between this instrumental form of mentoring and the more classical notions of the concept (East 1987) is particularly pertinent in nurse education. For Morton-Cooper & Palmer (1993) the notion of mentoring in nurse education as being merely support for tasks linked to professional and vocational qualification would fall into the category of 'pseudo or quasi-mentoring' because the focus is only on getting the qualifications, more akin to support provided by personal tutors. 'True mentoring' of a classical nature is reserved for the holistic support for the individual in the development of a new and complex professional role (see Fig. 8.2).

THE CONCEPTUAL BASES FOR MENTORING

Although there has been little systematic research into the conceptual bases for mentoring there is a considerable amount of published material on the subject. Gray & Gray (1986) and Noller & Frey (1983) provide bibliographies of studies of mentoring in academic settings, adult development programmes, career and business management, education, leadership training, medicine, nursing, psychotherapy and general supervisory/training programmes.

The concepts associated with mentoring are embedded within several theories of human learning and development. Thomas et al (1982) refer to three such theories in their examination of the conceptual base of mentoring:

- Life-span development—Erik Erikson.
- Stages of intellectual and ethical development—William Perry.
- Social learning theory—Albert Bandura.

LIFE-SPAN DEVELOPMENT

Erikson's (1969) model of life-span development describes a series of eight stages from birth to old age. Each stage has a 'psychosocial crisis' associated with it as shown in Table 8.2.

Erikson used this term to emphasise that the tasks to be completed are both psychological (in relation to the self) and social (in relation to others) and that there are important developmental issues to be resolved. The stages are age-linked but should not be construed as a series of steps leading to an 'achievement' within a given stage because each stage depends on the previous stages and affects the ones that follow. The outcome of each stage is dependent on the balance between an individual's positive and negative experiences and this tension remains throughout life.

The seventh stage (mid-adulthood) is the stage of most relevance for mentors. The central task of this stage, generativity versus stagnation, is dependent on the favourable outcomes of the preceding developmental tasks which are likely to give a person a basic trust in the world, hope for the future, a sense of confidence and purpose, and a successful pattern of relating to others. (See Box 8.1.)

The strengths of the generative person are 'production and care' so these represent core qualities for mentoring construed from Erikson's perspective. Thomas et al refer to the generative person as 'the perfect mentor' and Merriam (1983) claims that 'mentoring is one manifestation of this mid-life task'.

To be able to relate to and use a mentor effectively requires that the mentee is sufficiently mature emotionally to be able to receive support

Table 8.2   Implications of Erikson's eight life stages (adapted from Erikson 1985)

Stage	Age (approx)	Task	Favourable outcome	Unfavourable outcome	Lasting accomplishment of successful outcome
1	Infancy (0–1 year)	Basic trust v. mistrust	Feelings of being wanted and loved and cared for. A sense of stability and order in experience—the result of physical and emotional 'mothering'.	Life is chaotic and unconnected. Child likely to be psychologically and possibly physically disabled. Higher infant mortality than usual. Retardation, possibly autism.	Drive and hope
2	Toddler (1–3 years)	Autonomy v. shame and doubt	Learns to stand on own two feet. Feeds self and begins to control bodily functions and use language to meet basic needs. Learns to say and accept 'no' as well as 'yes'. Begins to learn rules of society.	Lack of autonomy, passive dependence on others. Unable to assert own will, resulting in over-obedience. Paradoxically, is unable to accept 'no' and so results in constantly rebellious personality, perhaps delinquency.	Self-control and will power
3	Pre-school (about 4–5 years)	Initiative v. guilt	Has developed memory, can go and come back, both in place and time. Starts to learn adult gender roles. More loving, cooperative, secure in family. Good chance of becoming able to make moral choices.	Always wants to be 'in control'. Sense of competition drives individual to be over-competitive. May be always outside the law.	Direction and purpose
4	School (about 6–12 years)	Industry v. inferiority	Learns the basic skills of society—the 'how to's, the 'three Rs'. Learns to feel worthy and competent.	If person fails to learn industry, begins to feel inferior compared with others. If over-learns industry, may become too task-oriented and over-conform to society.	Method and competence
5	Adolescence (age 12 to late teens or early adulthood)	Identity v. role confusion	Sexual maturation and sexual identity. Ponders question 'Who am I?' as distinct from family. Develops social friendships. Tends to reject and be in conflict with family. Begins to discover role in life.	May not achieve an identity separate from family. May not become socially adult or sexually stable.	Devotion and fidelity
6	Early adulthood	Intimacy v. isolation	Learns to share passions, interests, problems with another individual. Also relates to others at work, in community, as well as in family. Achieves stability.	Inability to be intimate with others. Becomes fixated at adolescent level, preoccupied with sensation-seeking and self-pleasure. Avoids responsibility and lacks stability.	Affiliation and love
7	Middle adulthood	Generativity v. self-absorption and stagnation	Fosters creativity and growth in others younger than self. Provides leadership, seeks to contribute to community, next generation, world. 'Minds the store'. May be most creative period of life.	Growth limited, remains rooted in past. Becomes 'cog-in-wheel', automated. May experience breakdown of zest for life. Feels life is passing him/her by.	Production and care
8	Old age	Ego integrity v. despair	Recognises and accepts diminishing faculties. Realises and faces own death. Feeling of having lived a 'good enough' life, paving the way for future generations. Dignity of truly 'wise' person.	Reaps bitter fruits of what was sown or not sown earlier. Fears death. An old age of misery, anxiety and despair.	Renunciation and wisdom

Box 8.1   Erikson's seventh stage of lifespan development

The generative person is able to foster creativity and growth in others. This may be the most creative period in a person's life, the culmination of a favourable enough outcome of the preceding stages leading to trust, stability, self-esteem, fidelity, competence, the capacity to work and have concern for others. From this solid foundation the generative person can provide leadership and contribute to the community, the next generation and the world at large.

In contrast, the opposite of generativity is self-absorption and stagnation. If preceding stages have resulted in a person feeling powerless, directionless, rootless and inferior, the capacity to feel concern for others is stunted.

without feeling crushed or overwhelmed by the difference in status and experience. This requires that the mentee has already established an adequate sense of identity and the ability to relate effectively to others i.e. to have a positive outcome from earlier tasks in stages 5 and 6. See Boxes 8.2 and 8.3 for a description of negative and positive experiences in mentoring.

Box 8.2   A negative experience of mentoring

Annie is a very highly qualified and experienced nurse tutor. She is the mentor to Lucy who is in her second year of training. Reflecting on her experience Annie says:
'I don't think I'm overstating to say that my mentee sees me as a minor irritation, a person who has very little more, if any more, expertise than she has. Lucy seems to think 'Here's someone who thinks she knows it all. If I want to get this qualification I suppose I've got to tolerate her and be civil but I won't go out of my way to draw on what she might be able to offer me because I don't believe she can offer me anything'. She is always reluctant to discuss assignment or project material with me although she's quite prepared to use me as a matter of convenience to deliver work for her. We don't have confrontations but I feel I'm there out of sheer forbearance on her part rather than a desire to achieve something together.'
Lucy finds it difficult to share herself with colleagues at work. She tends to keep herself to herself, feeling somewhat overwhelmed by intimate relationships and has problems with authority figures.
Lucy says 'I know vaguely what it means to have a mentor. If I require help I can chat with her. I don't have a great deal of contact with her actually; she's quite marginal. It's not negative, it's bland. I can take it or leave it.'

Box 8.3   A positive mentoring experience

Edwina is just two years from retirement after a successful career as a nurse practitioner. Ben is a nurse coming towards the end of his training.
Edwina says: 'You see a light at the end of the tunnel and it says retirement above the door and you're just pulling up the ladder to coast home when somebody like Ben comes along. I realise now I am a nurse to the day I retire. There's a lot for me to learn still and my patients benefit even though they never see Ben. I feel basically I am a support unit to the course but one step away from the course so Ben can come to me and explain what his basic problem is with less embarrassment than if he went to one of his tutors. Ben sometimes thinks his questions are stupid questions and they're not—they're very important questions. It reminds me, although I'm very experienced now, of the worries I had when I was a student. It's empathy really.'
Ben says: 'She provides me with a stabilising influence. I like her and I trust her. I feel she can hold a confidence and I have confidence in her. I can lean on her. I was afraid I would reveal too much of myself and she would get fed up with me. I think she's had a difficult role with me because I've been like a barrel of dynamite at times. She's actually handled it very well because she's let *me* work through it. She's got personal qualities in that she leads rather than drives and has this ability to go right to the heart of the matter. As a result when I'm floundering along…I suppose when we're floundering we're all embarrassed but I know she will be able to headline it, just little bits of help, just enough to lift me and carry me through. So I'm very happy with my mentor and I'm very aware of what it must feel like to be handling someone like me. I'm grateful to her. I don't know what else to say except to repeat that I'm grateful.'

INTELLECTUAL AND ETHICAL DEVELOPMENT

Perry (1981) is concerned to plot the normal expected change in individuals' intellectual and ethical development. In common with other stage theories, Perry's is hierarchical, though the time taken to pass through the stages will vary from individual to individual and the passage may stop or go into reverse, especially if external conditions become too threatening or over-whelming. The nine positions of Perry's scheme are grouped into four categories. (See Fig 8.3.)

The mentor's role begins functioning at position 9 when the mentoring relationship offered is likely to be characterised by independence, flexibility, openness and the ideal combination of

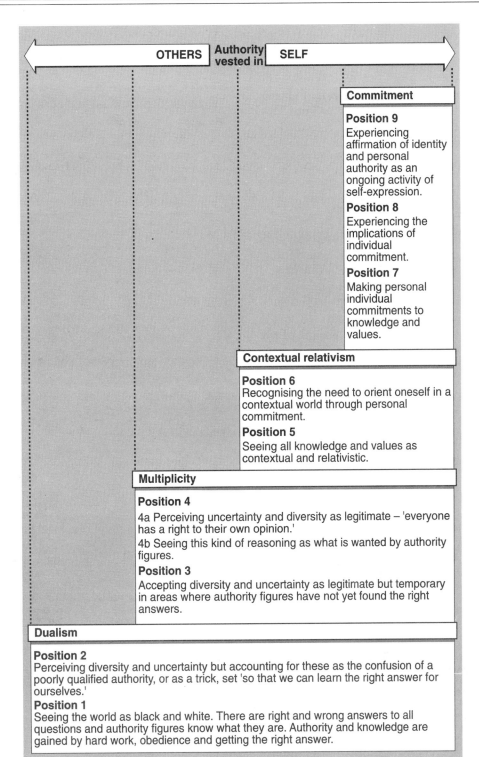

Figure 8.3   Perry's four stages of intellectual and ethical development

support and challenge. The novice in any situation, especially nursing, is likely to be operating at an earlier stage and so can potentially be aided in development by a mentor who 'knows the ropes' and has been through the earlier stages. How often the newcomer wants to know the 'right' way of doing something and, how difficult to realise that there may not be a 'right' way but rather a range of options from which the newcomer must choose.

SOCIAL LEARNING THEORY

Bandura's social learning theory is used to clarify an important aspect of mentoring i.e. modelling. If the mentor is perceived as a person worthy of emulation, the mentee is likely to imitate the mentor's behaviour, values and attitudes. Such imitation, or modelling, is likely to result from the whole integrated behaviour and actions of the mentor rather than just his words. The mentor might act as a model for the acquisition of complex social and interpersonal skills or, in a situation in which mistakes could be costly and dangerous, a model of safe, confident, clinical behaviour.

---

1. OBSERVATIONAL LEARNING

Modelling by imitating any form of behaviour desired by the imitator.

Models might be :

a. **An actual person**
   – peer, colleague, friend.
b. **A symbolic model**
   – fictional character, religious, mythical or legendary figure.
c. **An exemplary model**
   – parent, teacher, boss.

For example :

(a) Su-Lin wants to be as good a nurse as her colleague, Amy, whom she has worked alongside on her initial placement.
(b) Carlos has always found TV hospital dramas compulsive viewing. Now he wants to be a nurse just like his favourite character in a current serial.
(c) Both of David's parents have worked in medical settings and his ambition is to follow their example.

In Bandura's definition of modelling, imitation is seen as more than merely copying behaviour and is divided into three categories. (See Fig 8.4.)

---

2. INHIBITORY/DISINHIBITORY EFFECTS

Imitation of deviant behaviour may have :

a. **An inhibitory effect**
   – deviant behaviour is seen to be punished and therefore inhibited in the observer
b. **A disinhibitory effect**
   – deviant behaviour is seen not to be punished and is therefore imitated.

For example :

(a) Lottie observes her friend Irene being disciplined for her continual lateness for work. She makes her own decision to be punctual because she cannot bear the thought of being told off which for her would feel like a humiliation.
(b) Although Mark knows that he should respect confidential information about patients he has observed other staff leaving notes around the ward and that they don't get into trouble. This leads Mark to treat the patients' personal information carelessly and without respect.

---

3. ELICITING EFFECT

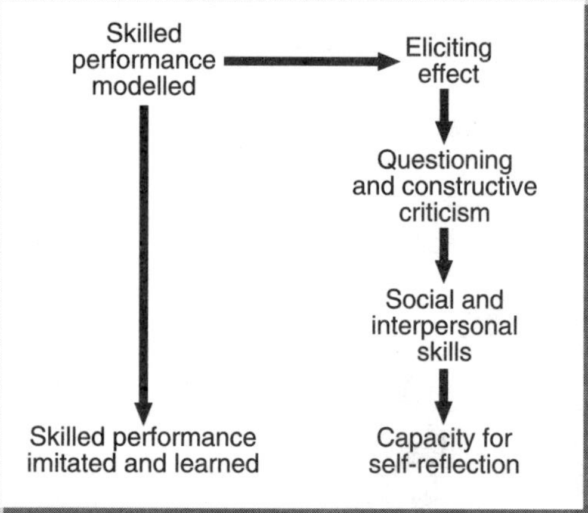

For example :

Helen is working on her geriatric placement. As she observes the staff bathing the patients she learns how to do this skilfully so that all of their physical needs are met. She also learns that there is a lot more to this job than just the physical aspects of care as she observes the great sensitivity, understanding and humour shown by the staff.

Figure 8.4 Bandura's three categories of learning by observation and imitation

It is important to note again that this social learning theory is based on operant conditioning (see Chapter 2) and is concerned with reinforcement and imitation principally in relation to behaviour control and modification.

Zey (1984) warns that to call the mentoring relationship role-modelling is to understate the power of the interaction. Referring to the process as 'role participation', a most potent form of learning, Zey claims that this is as different from role-modelling as on-the-job training is from text book learning. The mentee is not a passive observer but an active participant in the learning process, integrating observational learning into previous learning.

The common theme that runs throughout each of these three theories is that a healthy mentoring relationship is one where both mentor and mentee have a trusting attitude towards each other. The mentor is able to share ideas and opinions from a clearly articulated value framework, without imposing those ideas and opinions on the mentee. Generative people have the capacity for industry and competence and the ability and desire to foster these strengths in others.

MENTORING IN CONTEXT

Mentoring is a complex and dynamic process and can be implemented in a variety of ways, embracing both classical and instrumental mentoring. This section examines mentoring in the context of large organisations, education and nursing.

MENTORING IN ORGANISATIONS

In an organisational setting mentoring may take place within contractual relationships, which are initiated formally by the organisation in order to maintain its cohesion and stability. Within this setting mentoring is implemented as part of a programme of organisational or career development rather than personal adult development, although these are not mutually exclusive.

Large firms such as Shell, ICI, the Institute of Chartered Accountants, Local Authorities and Regional Health Authorities use mentoring as part of their management strategies. Mentoring may be formalised in order to benefit the company or institution or it might focus on new entrants and/or 'high flyers'. There are potential disadvantages in focusing mentoring programmes on a particular group, for example graduates, in that staff excluded from the mentoring programme may feel devalued, disadvantaged and demotivated in comparison.

The concept of mentoring in an organisational setting tends to involve what Zey has described as the 'mutual benefits model' in which the instrumental relationship concerned with the career development of the mentee is expanded to include possible benefits for the mentor, the mentee and the organisation as shown in Figure 8.5.

Problems in the mentoring relationship may arise between the mentor and mentee or between the mentoring pair and the organisation. Any difficulties within the mentor/mentee relationship may stem from poor communication, leading to a mismatch of perceptions, from a failure to communicate needs and goals or from overdependence. Problems arising between the mentoring pair and the organisation often include a failure on the mentor's part to assess the political environment accurately or an inability to control the political environment. Zey refers to the 'black halo' effect of a politically weak mentor 'contaminating' the mentee.

Whilst recognising mentoring as powerful in human resource development, mentoring should not be the only form of career development within an organisation. A variety of staff development and training opportunities is needed to avoid the dangers of elitism and consequent resentment and to avoid confusion caused by applying the term mentoring to induction programmes or specific short-term tasks.

MENTORING IN EDUCATION

Mentoring programmes are used in a wide variety of educational settings for example in programmes for gifted children; initial and in-service teacher training and staff development

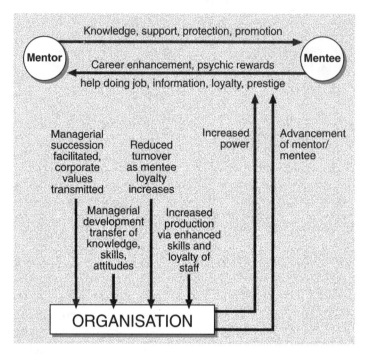

Figure 8.5   The mutual benefits of mentoring (adapted from Zey 1984)

programmes; undergraduate and faculty programmes; small business advice, cooperatives, adult and community programmes and in nurse education which is covered in more detail below. The aims of these programmes include the fostering of independent, self-managed learning; support for open learning projects; and the provision of learning experiences not possible in the classroom or lecture theatre.

Egan (1986) reports on North American State programmes which use 'master-teachers' as a source of support, advice and inspiration for new teachers. Referring to the difficulties during the first three years of teaching, Egan asks whether mentors could ease the transition from student to novice teacher to professional teacher. Teaching can be a 'professional desert' for new staff, with communication made difficult by the isolation of classroom experiences and a fear of discussing problems or asking too many questions because of the risk of appearing incompetent.

Teachers may need different types of mentoring at different points in their careers. The new teacher needs to deal with survival in the classroom; the more experienced teacher may

need discussion on the complex issues of education. Neil (1986) supports this progression of changing needs, referring to the teacher in the first year of teaching as being self-oriented; in the second and third years of teaching as being teacher-oriented; and in the fourth year as being pupil-centred. Mentoring programmes in education could form the basis of collaborative in-service training, and would be valuable for supportive work including mutual planning; demonstration of teaching techniques; structured feedback; developing strengths and skills and allowing risk-taking in a safe environment.

Egan refers to the many roles that mentors play in in-service training and claims that mentees speak glowingly about the opportunity to observe their mentors teaching. This is viewed as real opportunity to see theory being put into practice. (See Box 8.4.)

This form of role-modelling enables new teachers to observe some features of teaching that are difficult to learn in any other way. For example, 'student-centredness' and appropriate forms of communication and behaviour in the classroom might only be learned in this way.

Box 8.4 A teaching observation

'In lots of ways he was a classic person for me to have as a mentor because I've got a lot of respect for his track record. He's obviously been teaching a long time and watching him teach was quite an amazing experience. He has terrific humour, he's very approachable. There's a lot of laughter with him. He teaches very dry subjects but at the same time he has this ability to relate it to silly everyday events which are actually valid analogies. Being slightly ridiculous it makes the students laugh but at the same time they remember the concepts.'

MENTORING IN NURSING

The role of the mentor in nursing is currently being examined as part of the UKCC-initiated reforms which have had a profound effect on nursing and nurse education. The core studies component of Project 2000 comprises an ever-increasing body of knowledge and whilst this is important, there are aspects of nursing which require more than knowledge alone. For example, one has only to look at Clause 5 of the UKCC Code of Professional Conduct which stipulates that registered nurses, midwives and health visitors should 'work in a collaborative and cooperative manner with other health care professionals and recognise and respect their particular contribution within the health care team'.

The interpretation and application of this clause, and of the whole Code, can only be developed in the context of a collaborative and cooperative relationship with more experienced colleagues. The dynamic interplay of skills, knowledge, understanding, professional attitudes and values is embedded in the concept of the reflective practitioner.

The justification for mentoring programmes is that they offer an opportunity, rooted in the application of adult learning and developmental theories, to enable new entrants to nursing to make a smoother transition from novice to knowledgeable practitioner.

This argument has not been accepted in the profession without reservation. Questions about mentoring and whether nurses actually need mentors have been asked and the taken-for-granted acceptance of mentoring as intrinsically good and positive has also been questioned.

Examining gender influences and particularly the lack of role socialisation opportunities (the old-boy network) available to women, Campbell-Heider (1986) discusses the implications of applying traditional i.e. male/mentorship models in the predominantly female context of nursing. There are considerable differences between the application of more traditional male oriented mentoring—stressing sponsorship and advancement of the individual—and mentoring programmes in nursing. Aspiring nurse managers, administrators and educators, however, may well prefer a more traditional relationship, seeking career advice and sponsorship in addition to support and intellectual stimulation.

The first reference to mentors, as part of course approval processes, was made by the ENB circular (1987/28/MAT) which defined a mentor as 'an appropriately qualified and experienced first level nurse/midwife/health visitor who, by example and facilitation, guides, assists and supports the student in learning new skills, adopting new behaviours and acquiring new attitudes'.

This reference is clearly linked to Clause 12 of the UKCC Code of Professional Conduct which states: 'in the context of the individual's own knowledge, experience and sphere of authority, (the nurse should) assist peers and subordinates to develop professional competence in accordance with their needs'. This has not, however, led to clarity and congruence regarding the role and function of mentors within nursing.

Research and mentoring

Although American experiences are often quoted as the source of mentoring initiatives in Great Britain, questions about their effectiveness are also asked in the United States. Surveying the American scene, Hagerty (1986) provides a critical analysis of mentoring literature and examines the concept and theory, basic assumptions, related research, and the resulting generalisations and implications. Cautious and sceptical about some of the more florid claims made in support of mentoring from earlier studies, Hagerty points out that these assertions have been laid on weak foundations. Some studies confused their definition of mentor by including it in a range of supportive roles; others did not include any definition at all.

The samples used for research on mentoring have been small, selective, atypical and non-random. There has been little use of control groups and research methods have tended to be descriptive, retrospective and anecdotal. Thus, conclusions and implications based on existing research are likely to be unsupported and inappropriate. Hagerty further claims that research studies have too often been merely a description of activities and there has been confusion about whether it is the person or the process, the purposes or the activities which are being described.

There have been many assumptions made about mentoring and although these are sometimes unexamined they are often presented as facts. Common assumptions include the belief that having a mentor is a requisite for success and that is why women do not succeed; that the only success that counts is upward mobility through the organisational hierarchy; and that mentoring is the same across all work settings.

In Britain, concerns have been expressed about the absence of a clear definition of mentoring (Morle 1990, Armitage & Burnard 1991). These authors go on to introduce the idea of 'precep-torship'—an individual teaching/learning method in which students are assigned to 'preceptors' who act as clinical role models—as an alternative for helping to bridge the theory/ practice gap. Anforth (1992) reviews these arguments in her own clarification of the mentoring role and concludes that it should be retained in addition to the roles of preceptor, facilitator and assessor.

Assessment and mentoring

Mentoring programmes in nurse education highlight perhaps more sharply than in other settings the question of whether the role of mentor should include an assessment function. Can a mentor also act as assessor when he is perhaps working with, and helping, students who may be fearful of those with power? In this situation adult students might mask their anxieties and uncertainties with bravado if they fear that expressing uncertainty could affect their assessments.

Anforth, together with Morton-Cooper & Palmer, stresses the benefits of developing rapport between mentor and mentee, ideally in a continuous relationship which lasts throughout the training period, and the need for this to be separated from assessment procedures. This approach is much disputed. For example, describing the Torbay mentoring scheme, Morris et al (1988) include the assessment role as one of four main mentoring roles: role model/facilitator/ supervisor/assessor. They see the mentor as the 'obvious candidate' to be the student's assessor.

In the Torbay scheme the mentors, all RMNs, are given a week's training and are audited on their skills in mentoring. Learners are allocated to mentors on the basis of these audited skills rather than clinical areas. The average time spent in a mentoring relationship is 6 months and the mentor acts as an 'enabler/catalyst'. Morris et al do not advocate an 'inseparable bonding', instead they envisage a tripartite relationship between learner, mentor and tutor.

Potential/transitional space

Even though the nursing profession is constantly being redefined, it still demands certainty in many areas, particularly clinical areas. It may be difficult to incorporate models of training that allow for individual interpretation of an abstract, some would say slippery and elusive, concept such as mentoring. Some staff will need clarity imposed from the outside, others will feel comfortable in determining their own clarity. If nursing is claiming the title of profession then staff must be prepared for a role which incor-porates and encourages autonomy.

The changes in nurse education herald a period of transition. Institutions must manage transitions efficiently if they are to survive. Learning that takes place during such periods might be compared with Winnicott's (1982) ideas on transitional phenomena, which are concentrated in the space between inner and outer experiences.

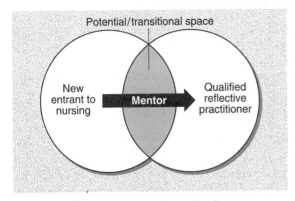

Figure 8.6   The area of potential/transitional space

It is in this 'potential space' that children learn to play and, if they are fortunate, continue to do so throughout their lives in active, exploratory learning which enables them to create their own understanding and insight. This idea lies at the heart of student-centred learning. Mentoring takes place within the potential space between two people. The result is the outcome of what they are able to create together (see Fig. 8.6).

Mentoring programmes need to encompass not only the development of competent clinical nurses but also the development of an individual's ability to become self-directing and thoughtful—the reflective practitioner.

SO WHAT IS A MENTOR?

The research into the conceptual bases for mentoring and its application in organisational, educational and nursing settings reveals the complexity of the role of a mentor. Cross (1976) reviewed the skill classifications in the US Dictionary of Occupational titles and found that mentoring was listed as the most complex role in terms of required interpersonal skills.

This complexity has led to a failure by some researchers to conceptualise the role. There has also been a variety of uses of the word mentor so that the definition varies from study to study. Mentoring is too complex for an adequate description through the use of a single procedure.

Given this complexity it is not surprising that research into the application of mentoring in organisational, educational and nursing settings has tended to break the concept down into its functional components. In nursing this has led to confusion about the nature of mentoring and the similarities and differences between this and preceptorship and tutoring.

It may be worth distinguishing between the need to get the 'right' definition and the need to have a 'clear' definition. The classical interpretation of the role leads us into metaphor and thence into personal interpretation. The desire for a clear definition of the role may indicate difficulty in coping with the tension of a complex, interpersonal role rooted in subjective experience. This tension may be resolved by resorting to an operational definition and being prescriptive about what a mentor is expected to do. There will always be differences in personal interpretation of the role: sometimes a nurse mentor will be a classical mentor; sometimes an instrumental mentor.

The development of appropriate interpersonal skills is highly important to the success of a mentoring relationship characterised by an interactional dialogue, shared problem solving and mutual exploration. These skills have a broad overlap with the skills of counselling described in Chapter 9.

If mentoring is construed as a bridging process between theory and practice it can serve several levels of activity, spanning not only induction and initial training but also continuing professional development for practitioners and managers. The stronger the bridge, the more confident the mentoring pair and the more frequent the journeys across the bridge, backwards and forwards, from not knowing to knowing, from not understanding to understanding, in an on-going process until eventually theory becomes integrated into practice. As a result of being mentored it is hoped that the mentee will become an autonomous professional who is self-reflective and self-directing.

Mentoring is not something that is given or done to others, it is about the relationships between people. What distinguishes fine mentors is their capacity and willingness to care. They know that they exist as mentors only because they are part of a relationship.

REFERENCES

Anforth P 1992 Mentors, not assessors. Nurse Education 1992. 12:299-302.

Armitage P, Burnard P 1991 Mentors or preceptors? Narrowing the theory practice gap. Nurse Education Today, 11: 223-229.

Bandura A 1977 Social learning theory. Englewood Cliffs, Prentice Hall, New Jersey.

Bandura A , Walters R H 1963 Social learning and personality development. Holt, Rinehart & Winston, New York.

Campbell-Holder N 1986 Do nurses need mentors? Image 183:110-113.

Clutterbuck D 1985 Everybody needs a mentor: how to foster talent within the organisation. IPM.

Cross K P 1976 Accent on learning, improving instruction and re-shaping the curriculum. Jossey Bass, San Francisco.

Daloz L A 1986 Effective teaching and mentoring: realising the transformational power of adult learning experiences. Jossey-Bass, San Francisco.

East P I 1987 The mentoring relationship. Unpublished MA thesis. University of Loughborough.

Egan J B 1986 Characteristics of classroom teachers mentor-protege relationships. In: Gray W, Gray M M 1986 Mentoring: an aid to excellence, Vol. I, International Association.

Erikson E 1969 Childhood and society, 2nd edn. New York, Norton.

Gray W A, Gray M M 1986 A comprehensive annotated bibliography of important references. International Association for Mentoring, Vancouver, Canada.

Gray W A, Gray M M 1986 Mentoring: aid to excellence. Proceedings of the 1st International Conference on Mentoring, vols I and II. International Association for Mentoring, Vancouver, Canada.

Hagerty B 1986 A second look at mentors. Nursing Outlook 34 1:16-24

Kegan R 1982 The evolving self. London, Harvard University Press.

Levinson D 1978 The seasons of a man's life. New York, Alfred Knopf.

Merriam S S 1983 Mentors and Proteges: A critical review of the literature in Adult Education Quarterly. Spring 1983 161-173.

Morle K M 1990 Mentorship—is it a case of the emperor's new clothes or a rose by any other name? Nurse Education Today 10(1)66-69 Longman Group.

Morris N, John G, Keen T 1988 Mentors: learning the ropes. Nursing Times 84 46:24-27.

Morton-Cooper A, Palmer A 1993 Mentoring and preceptorship. Blackwell Scientific, Oxford.

Neil R 1986 Current models and approaches to in-service teacher education. In: Brit J of In-service Education Vol 12, no. 2, 58-67.

Noller R B, Frey B 1983 Mentoring: an annotated bibliography. New York, Brearly Ltd.

Perry W G 1981 Cognitive and ethical growth: the making of meaning. In: Chickering A E 1981 The Modern American College. Jossey-Bass, San Francisco.

Rowntree D 1981 A dictionary of education. Harper & Row, London.

Thomas R, Murrell P H, Chickering A W 1982 Theoretical bases and feasibility issues for mentoring and developmental transcripts. In: Brown R D, De Coster D A (eds) 1982 See Further Reading.

Winnicott D W 1982 The maturational processes and the facilitating environment: studies in the theory of emotional development. London, The Hogarth Press Ltd., and the Institute of Psycho-Analysis.

Zey M G 1984 The mentor connection. Dow Jones Irwin, Illinois.

FURTHER READING

Baker S 1990 The key to nurse education. Nursing Standard, 4:39-43.

Brown R D, De Coster D A (eds) 1982 Mentoring transcript systems for promoting student growth. In: New directions for student services No 19. San Francisco, Jossey Bass.

Butterworth T, Faugier J 1992 Clinical supervision and mentorship in nursing. Chapman & Hall, London

Donovan J 1990 The concept and role of mentor. Nurse Education Today, 10 (4) 294-298.

Knowles M 1973 The adult learner: a neglected species. Gulf Publishing Company, Houston.

Knowles M 1986 Using Learning contracts. Jossey-Bass, San Francisco.

Kram E K 1988 Mentoring at work: developmental relationships in organisational life. University Press of America,Lanham,USA.

Monaghan J, Lunt N 1992 Mentoring: person process practice and problems. B.J.Educ.Studies No 3.

Rogers C R 1951 Client centred therapy. Houghton, Boston.

Rogers C R 1969 Freedom to learn. Merrill, Columbus Ohio.

Rogers C R 1974 On becoming a person. Constable, London.

Rothera M et al 1991 The role of subject mentor in further education. British Journal of In-service Education Vol 17 No 2:126-137.

Speizer J J 1981 Role models, mentors and sponsors: The elusive concepts in signs: Journal of Women in Culture and Society Vol 6, No 4, 1981.

Talbert E G, Phelps M S 1986 Technical skills of mentoring: a training module for teacher mentors. A paper presented to the 1st International Conference on Mentoring, 24th July 1986, Vancouver, Canada.

Tough A 1979 The adult's learning projects 2nd edn. Ontario Institute for Studies in Education, Toronto.

Wrightsman L S 1981 Research methodologies for assessing mentoring. A paper presented to the Annual meeting of the American Psychological Association, Los Angles, August 1981. In: Gray W, Gray M M A Comprehensive annotated bibliography of important references.

International Association for Mentoring, Vancouver, Canada.

9

The counselling relationship

Andy Betts

INTRODUCTION

Most nurses and midwives are *not* counsellors but are professional helpers whose work includes, to a greater or lesser extent, providing psychological support to people who are experiencing a diversity of personally significant life events. This specific type of communication forms the focus for this chapter which examines the nature of the counselling relationship.

There is some evidence to suggest that many nurses have difficulty in establishing and maintaining a facilitative relationship (Macleod Clark 1985, Burnard & Morrison 1991). This chapter looks at the principles of counselling which the health carer may apply to help her become more effective at establishing, maintaining and ending a facilitative relationship. It also recognises the importance of developing the ability to continually reflect on these interpersonal encounters. It is hoped that the issues raised will promote a re-evaluation of the reader's own experiences and a clearer sense of purpose, intention and direction in this type of helping.

CLARIFYING THE TERMINOLOGY

Harris (1987) notes that counselling has become a vogue term with a broad populist meaning covering a range of different activities. In contrast to this general meaning, counselling today has a more precise definition within a confined and specialist arena. The counselling movement in the

United Kingdom has evolved over the past 30 years to be gradually accepted as a profession that is shaking off a lingering image of well-meaning, untrained do-gooders. Counsellors now have an established professional body—the British Association of Counselling (BAC)—which is energetic in debating and establishing accredited standards of practice and training for counsellors. It is largely due to these efforts that the term counselling has come to mean a more specialist form of helping. Despite this maturation, Howard (1988) questions whether it is possible to write a definition of counselling which is not 'banal, question-begging or vacuous'. The BAC (1990) defines counselling as:

the skilled and principled use of relationship to facilitate self-knowledge, emotional acceptance and growth, and the optimal development of personal resources. Counselling may be concerned with: addressing and resolving specific problems, making decisions, coping with crisis, working through feelings of inner conflict, or improving relationships with others. The counsellor's role is to facilitate the client's work in ways that respect the client's values, personal resources and capacity for self-determination.

(BAC 1990)

This somewhat lengthy definition is the result of much debate and serves to illustrate the difficulties of pinning down what the activity of counselling is in a precise sense. Some of the misunderstandings associated with the term counselling are illustrated by Box 9.1.

Box 9.1 Commonly held myths about counselling

1. Counselling is predominantly concerned with giving advice.
2. Counselling is just common sense—we do it anyway.
3. Counselling is to do with discipline.
4. All health carers are trained in this work.
5. Counselling is by nature vague, unstructured and lacking direction.
6. People can profitably be 'sent' for counselling.
7. Nurses do not have time for counselling.
8. Counselling is about talking, not action.

There is often confusion regarding the respective meanings of such terms as counselling, use of counselling skills and psychotherapy. This confusion is illustrated in the case of health care workers:

Box 9.2 Counselling or the use of counselling skills?

Kathy, a staff nurse on a children's ward listens skilfully to the mother of a 5-year-old child who has been admitted for minor surgery. Kathy allows the mother to express her fears about the operation without intruding or belittling them. In everything that she does and says Kathy demonstrates genuine concern for the mother as she tries to understand from her perspective.

At this time is Kathy engaged in listening skills or counselling skills or counselling, and does it matter? The BAC (1990) states clearly that unless both the user and recipient explicitly contract to enter into a counselling relationship then the helper is using counselling skills rather than counselling. If we observed Kathy in both a contracted and non-contracted counselling relationship, she may do the same thing in both situations. Therefore, an important distinction is whether the counselling is explicit or not. In this example if Kathy and the mother had not openly contracted counselling then Kathy was using counselling skills rather than counselling. For most health carers in the majority of situations this is likely to be the case.

To complicate matters further it can be argued that the skills Kathy demonstrates are not exclusively 'counselling skills' but are inter-personal or communication skills which are widely applicable in many other contexts for many different purposes (Bond 1989). Certainly the skills learned in becoming a counsellor are lifeskills in as much as they equip the individual for most other human encounters. Perhaps there is no clear demarcation between these various activities and, as suggested by Pratt (1990), the differences being searched for are more to do with the definition of roles than those of practice.

The ethical importance of this discussion is to protect the client by ensuring that they are not exploited, deceived or harmed by individuals who do not realise, or who choose to deny, their own limitations. In addition, unless helpers are sure about what it is they are engaged in, how will they know how effective they are?

Counselling and advice

Counselling and giving advice are different types of helping. Advice is given from the helper's frame of reference but counselling is firmly grounded within the client's frame of reference. Advice giving is more directive and consequently takes away some of the self-responsibility of the client. Most counselling approaches are less directive and serve to empower clients to help themselves. Both types of helping have a place in nursing but the wise nurse knows clearly when advice is appropriate and when to use counselling skills.

Counselling and psychotherapy

A long-running debate continues on whether a difference exists between counselling and psychotherapy and if so, what it is and is it helpful? There is a growing consensus that the terms may be used interchangeably in most cases (Patterson 1986). However, there may be extremes at either end of the spectrum that could not be readily described as one or the other (see Fig. 9.1). Psychotherapy, for instance, is rarely brief in duration whereas counselling is often short-term and may comprise only a few agreed sessions. At the other end of the spectrum, a person attending sessions three times per week for several years and focusing on reconstructive work is unlikely to define this as counselling but as psychotherapy.

So where does this discussion take us and how may it shed light on an understanding of the counselling relationship in the context of health care?

Confusion about the term counselling probably exists because of the word's historical associations. The term 'to counsel' has been interpreted by many as a catch-all verb covering a whole range of human interactions. Over recent years the definition of counselling has evolved to mean a more specific helping activity. While these two distinct uses of the term co-exist confusion is likely to remain. However, the principles examined in this chapter have some application for all nurses in whatever context because they are engaged in what is essentially a helping and interpersonal process. A minority of nurses who have appropriate qualifications may use more formal counselling in their work but only when this is openly contracted with the client.

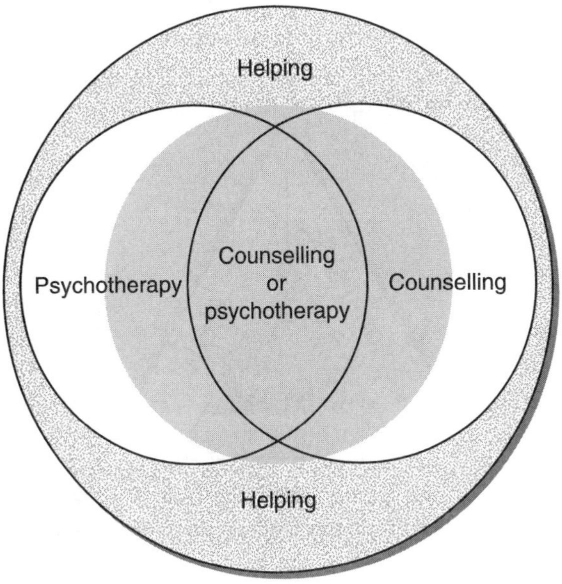

THE COUNSELLING RELATIONSHIP

AIMS

Counselling comprises hundreds of different approaches with widely contrasting views. Nevertheless, all these approaches share a broadly common aim i.e. to lead to valued outcomes in the client's day-to-day life. The counselling relationship is not an end in itself but a means to an end. Much as we all seem to value the attention and understanding of another individual this should not be the primary reason for counselling. The counselling relationship is only effective to the degree that it translates into more effective living on the part of the client. As a direct result of the counselling relationship something should happen outside of it. Egan (1990 p.7) notes:

Figure 9.1

effective helping results in something valued being in place that was not in place before the helping session(s): unreasonable fears will disappear or diminish to manageable levels; self confidence will replace self-doubt; addiction will be conquered; an operation will be faced with a degree of equanimity; a better job will be found; a new life will be breathed into a marriage; self-respect will be restored.

(Egan 1990)

This does not mean that the counselling relationship always ends with the client riding off into the sunset, all dreams fulfilled. Indeed, often the client's experience is a painful and demanding one but the ultimate aim is an improved quality of life. The emphasis of the relationship is concerned with helping the client to manage problems and develop unused opportunities towards living more resourcefully. The goal is not for the health carer to 'solve' the problem for the client but to provide the structure in which the individual is able to do the work and resolve the conflict in her own way.

To some extent this may cause dissonance for professional carers. There is evidence to suggest that health care professions have a history of taking away responsibility from the client/patient (Stimson & Webb 1975). The counselling relationship involves holding back on doing some of the things that carers do as part of their wider role. The wise adage applies that if you give a man fish he eats for the day; if you teach him to fish he eats for life. In other words, if you provide the space in which clients are able to help themselves they may not need future assistance because they have increased their own personal resources. In

this context a secondary aim of the health carer in the counselling relationship is to do themselves out of a job! Helpers should not be in the business of maintaining dependence but of empowering others to live more resourcefully and independently. In this sense the relationship is a collaborative partnership which has the client's self-responsibility as a core value.

THE NATURE OF THE RELATIONSHIP

Being with others

The principles of counselling are illustrated in Figure 9.2. The inner triangle contains the client and represents two important points. First, that the relationship is client-centred in the sense that the helper is there for the client in an unambiguous way. The relationship is very different to everyday encounters because the helper is there for the client—the dialogue is concentrated primarily on the thoughts, feelings and behaviours of the client. Most other human interactions are characterised by a more symmetrical exchange of mutual interests. Mearns & Thorne (1988 p.5) underline the principle that counselling is a pursuit of the subjective reality of

---

Box 9.3 Aims of the counselling relationship

1. To enable others to live more satisfying lives.
2. To provide an environment which helps others to help themselves.
3. To empower others to live more resourcefully and independently.
4. To assist others to manage their problems.
5. To help others to develop their unused resources and opportunities.
6. To enable others to come to terms with changed circumstances.

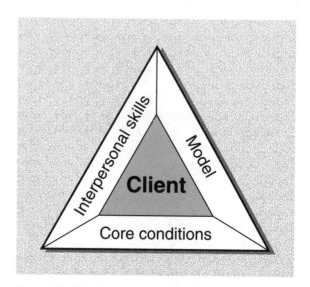

Figure 9.2 Principles of the counselling relationship

the client: 'High value is placed on the experience of the individual human being and on the importance of his or her subjective reality.'

Second, the helper holds and contains the structure and space in which the client does the work. The helper, represented by the external triangle of the diagram, contracts to hold a safe space for the client, represented by the inner triangle. This space consists of more than just the physical environment in which the counselling takes place. It also refers to a therapeutic space which represents a 'safe island' that is distinct from the rest of the client's experience. This space has clear boundaries that are established and maintained by the helper. The client experiences the helper as strong enough to both protect these boundaries and to not be overwhelmed by what the client brings to the session. Put simply, the helper is responsible for the process and the client for the content.

It is not coincidental that the core conditions form the base of the triangle. They are the foundations on which the counselling relationship is established, maintained and ended. Counselling is often described as a way of *being* with another person rather than a series of behaviours. This emphasis on the values of the relationship has much of its origin in the work of the humanist psychologist Carl Rogers (1951,

1967). He focused more on the qualities of the relationship itself than on the strategies, skills, techniques, models and frameworks being used by the helper. There is general agreement with Rogers' view (1967) that these core conditions are a necessary requisite for meaningful helping to take place but less consensus regarding his belief that they were sufficient in themselves.

Activity 9.1

Examine the ten questions posed by Rogers (Box 9.4). How many are you able to honestly answer in the affirmative in the context of your own helping relationships?

The challenge of exhibiting these values with all clients in all counselling relationships appears daunting (see Box 9.4). Rogers (1967) acknowledges that these qualities are ideals for which the helper continually strives rather than consistently achievable standards. All of these core conditions exist on a continuum rather than an 'all or nothing basis'. The life-long task for the helper is to continually strive to establish

---

Box 9.4 How can I create a helping relationship? (Rogers 1967)

1. Can I *be* in some way which will be perceived by the other person as trustworthy, dependable or consistent in some deep sense?
2. Can I be expressive enough as a person that what I am will be communicated unambiguously?
3. Can I let myself experience positive attitudes toward this other person—attitudes of warmth, caring, interest and respect?
4. Can I be strong enough as a person to be separate from the other?
5. Am I strong enough within myself to permit this person her separateness—can I permit her to be what she is?
6. Can I let myself enter fully into the world of her feelings and personal meanings and see them as she does?
7. Can I be acceptant of each facet of this other person which she presents to me?
8. Can I act with sufficient sensitivity in the relationship that my behaviour will not be perceived as threat?
9. Can I free her from the threat of external evaluation?
10. Can I meet this other individual as a person who is in the process of becoming, or will I be bound by her past and by my past?

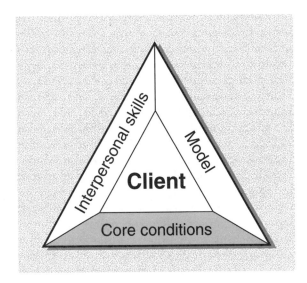

Figure 9.3 Core conditions

relationships based on these core conditions while acknowledging the reality that she will fall short of maintaining these conditions in all helping encounters. The core conditions consist of empathy, genuineness, respect, and confidentiality.

Empathy

Empathy is often seen as the most critical ingredient of the helping relationship. Carkhuff (1970) argues that without empathy there is no basis for helping. Kalisch (1971) defines empathy as 'the ability to sense the client's world as if it were your own, but without losing the *as if* quality' (Kalisch 1971 p.203).

This short definition contains some complex ideas. Empathic understanding is often described as 'standing in somebody else's shoes' but this is not the full story. Imagine how you might feel at the end of a day if you stood in the shoes of each person you meet in your helping role—experiencing their thoughts and feelings. Empathy involves retaining your own separateness while trying to understand the world from the other person's perspective. In order to do this it is necessary to understand the client's world *as if* you were inside it, attempting to see it with the client's eyes but keeping in touch with your own world. In this way the helper remains in a position to help—to get close enough to the client's experience to make a difference whilst retaining a sense of objectivity in order to hold on to the process and not become overwhelmed.

Empathy is different from sympathy—consider the example in Box 9.5.

The second response stays with Claire's experience in that it more accurately expresses what she feels and does not attempt to deny the emotional pain. It is likely that Claire would feel understood and continue to talk about her experience. This is probably more helpful for her than the initial response which is aimed at making Claire feel better in the short-term and illustrates the difference between sympathy and empathy. If empathy is the primary ingredient of effective helping (Carkhuff 1970, La Monica et al 1976, Truax & Mitchell 1971) it is not unreasonable to

---

Box 9.5 Empathy with the client

Claire lives in a house with three other women. Despite the fact that they all have some learning disabilities they are able to live reasonably independently. John, a community nurse, visits on a regular basis mainly to help the women with day-to-day management of the house and to offer support and encouragement. John has recently been working with Claire in helping her to develop more social contacts outside of the house. She had set herself the goal of attending a local church house group for the first time. During John's subsequent visit the conversation goes as follows:
Claire: (very upset) '*I'm really disappointed—I was too scared to go. I just couldn't face it.*'
John: (reassuring voice tone) '*Never mind. There's always next week. You will be feeling better by then*'.
John's response comes from a position of caring and goodwill but is sympathetic rather than empathetic. He fails to acknowledge Claire's disappointment and speaks from a position of optimistic hope rather than reflecting the reality of Claire's disappointment. A more empathetic and skilled response might be:
John: (concerned expression) '*This was so important for you and now you feel upset that you couldn't go through with it*'.

---

expect to see it widely demonstrated in the helping professions. You may decide for yourself whether or not this is the case but there are many reasons why it may not be (see Box 9.6).

It is important that helpers not only understand from the client's perspective but actively communicate that understanding to the client through the use of skilled communication. In this sense empathy involves both an attitude and a behavioural component. Helpers enter the client's world through attending, observing, listening and then convey that understanding through responding skills. How much of this core condition relates to an attitude and how much to skills is open to debate. It appears that empathic understanding may be increased by teaching the appropriate skills but it is less clear to what extent an empathic attitude or trait is influenced by educational experiences (Reynolds 1987). Clearly the early emotional experience of earlier relationships with other people will have a significant effect on the individual's ability to understand the world of others. The healthy psychosocial development of a child involves a

Box.9.6 Possible reasons for lack of empathy

1. Helpers may 'contaminate' clients' stories with their own experiences i.e. distort the client's reality because of their own similar experiences.
2. Helpers may make assumptions about clients' experiences that are unsubstantiated—filling in gaps rather than checking out the facts.
3. Helpers may fail to hear the 'music behind the words'—failing to pick up on some of the more subtle cues (often unspoken).
4. Helpers may not have developed the empathic listening and responding skills necessary to understand and convey that understanding to the client.
5. Helpers may lose concentration or be distracted.
6. Helpers may consciously choose not to hear certain things for fear of being overwhelmed.
7. Helpers may track their own lines of interest rather than staying with what the client sees as important.
8. Helpers may rush to move the conversation along rather than acknowledge what has been said.
9. Helpers may pretend to understand rather than check out what the reality is.
10. Helpers may too readily interpret clients' experiences or give advice from their own frame of reference.
11. Helpers may be sympathetic rather than empathetic.
12. Helpers may be judgemental or biased in their responses to clients.
13. Helpers may take over the conversation by talking about their own experiences, thoughts and feelings.

Box 9.7 Genuineness and helping (Egan 1990)

1. Do not over emphasise the helping role.
2. Be spontaneous but tactful i.e. not over-inhibited but sensitive.
3. Avoid defensiveness e.g. in response to negative criticism.
4. Be consistent.
5. Be open.
6. Work at being comfortable with behaviour that helps clients—e.g. not too relaxed or too uptight.

Relating deeply to others is a part of the effective helper's lifestyle rather than a role which is taken on and off. Inauthentic helping may appear as 'plastic counselling', or cloned behaviour learned from a counselling trainer or textbook where helpers mechanistically use behaviours and responses that disguise their own integrity, personality and communication style. It is those very qualities that make the helper unique as an individual which serve the relationship. The nurse who switches into 'helping mode' upon the sight of an individual in distress may be perceived by the client as patronising and untrustworthy.

Egan (1990) identifies six principles in relation to genuineness (Box 9.7).

Respect

Respect has been described as the deepest human need (Harre 1980). It is difficult to define what is meant by the term. Everyday use of the word tends to be conditional on qualities, attributes or behaviours of others. A person's professionalism, intelligence or skills may be highly respected. The inference being that if the person stopped displaying that aspect of themselves the respect for her may lessen. In the helping context respect is used in a more unconditional sense. Egan (1990 p. 65) defines respect as 'prizing people simply because they are human'. The suggestion is that respect remains consistent and is not influenced by the other person's thoughts, feelings and behaviours. The client's lifestyle may differ considerably from that of the helper and may sometimes clash with the helper's values but the effective helper recognises these differences and does not judge the client for them. This non-

gradual abandonment of an egocentric view of the world to be replaced by an acknowledgement of the different subjective experiences of others. If the developing child is unable to achieve this transition it is likely to be difficult for her to empathise with others in later life.

Genuineness

This is sometimes referred to as congruence or authenticity. All three of these terms refer to the helper being consistently real in the helping relationship. Corey (1986) suggests that congruent helpers are without a false front and that their inner experience matches their outer expression of that experience and vice versa. In other words what clients see is who the helper really is.

Box 9.8 Respect

Anna is the named nurse for Robert, a 30-year-old man admitted to the Acute Mental Health Unit with depression. Anna knows that in the past Robert has sexually abused his 7-year-old daughter. When she is with him she feels a sense of disgust and anger that he could have done such a thing. She works hard not to let this show but realises that because of her feelings she is unable to establish a therapeutic relationship with him. She talks to a colleague about the situation and together they decide that it is inappropriate for Anna to continue to be the named nurse. They discuss ways in which the situation could be handled sensitively without Robert experiencing it as rejection.

---

judgemental attitude to the client helps provide a relationship which feels safe, warm and accepting. Once again this presents a difficult challenge to the helper. From an early age individuals are socialised into making judgements about others—'I like him; I don't like her; I don't want anything to do with him unless he...'. A helping relationship requires the helper to suspend this type of critical judgement. If the helper is unable to do so then in all probability she is unable to help that individual and is unlikely to be the most suitable person to continue. Acknowledgement of this represents a strength rather than a failure and requires self-awareness, honesty and sensitivity. (See Box 9.8.)

If Anna had not addressed her own strong feelings and continued to work with Robert it is unlikely that she would have been much help to him. She found it difficult to see past Robert the abuser and was consequently unable to empathise with him. Many people in Anna's position would have experienced similar feelings to a greater or lesser extent. The important point is that she was able to recognise that this was seriously affecting Robert's care and that she had the courage to address this. Unconditional respect does not mean that the helper condones the client's behaviour but that she is not there to judge him for it.

Confidentiality

Confidentiality is a fundamental feature of the counselling relationship. Understandably people

are unlikely to confide in others unless they have some expectation that what they disclose will go no further. The counselling relationship by its very nature is confidential. On the surface this seems a reasonable premise for the nurse using counselling skills. In practice there are limits to the helper's responsibility in this respect. A nurse using counselling skills as a part of her role is still guided by the Professional Code of Conduct of the nurses' professional body (UKCC) in relation to confidentiality. If a client is in danger of harming herself or others then the nurse has a duty to break confidence. Dryden & Feltham (1992) stress that the counsellor should make the client aware of the nature and limits of confidentiality at the outset of counselling. This may seem an awkward thing to do for fear of alarming the client but the alternatives could be more difficult to manage.

Consider the following example (Box 9.9.):

Box 9.9 Confidentiality

Richard, a community psychiatric nurse (CPN) has been visiting Caroline a 33-year-old woman who was referred to the community mental health team by her General Practitioner because she was depressed. In previous meetings with Caroline, Richard had not explicitly mentioned confidentiality in their relationship. Caroline has grown to trust him and assumes that what she tells him is confidential. During a home visit she hesitantly discloses that she has been experiencing suicidal thoughts over the past week. She asks that he does not say anything to the doctor because she is afraid he will admit her to hospital. Richard's assessment is that Caroline is at risk of harming herself and that he has no option but to reveal this information to the doctor even though he realises that this may damage their relationship. He is honest but sensitive in explaining that he is unable to keep this information to himself and although Caroline is at first upset, no lasting damage is done to the helping relationship.

It is important that helpers are clear about the nature, purpose and limitations of confidentiality in their work and they are not misleading in the messages that they give to the client in this respect.

COUNSELLING AS A SKILLED ACTIVITY

Whilst the core conditions are the foundation of the counselling relationship this type of helping also involves socially skilled behaviours or interpersonal skills (Fig. 9.4). There is a risk that interpersonal skills may be over-emphasised in the sense that they are seen as the helping process itself rather than as at the service of the process. Counselling is much more than the application of a range of skills (Johnson & Heppner 1989). If helping is reduced to a series of microskills used in a disjointed or artificial manner then it is likely to be ineffective. Bond (1989) argues that it is when these interpersonal skills are laden with the values of counselling that they may be seen as counselling skills.

Helpers who are able to establish a relationship based on the core conditions will be more effective if they are competent in the use of interpersonal skills. The aim is to integrate the skills into one's own style of communicating so that they become natural rather than mechanistic. Chapter 5 addresses some of the issues involved in learning these interpersonal skills. Effective helpers continually reflect on their use of skills

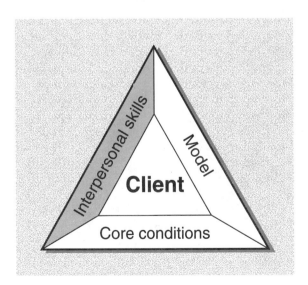

Figure 9.4 Counselling as a skilled activity

and understand that they can always improve the way in which they use them. An in-depth summary of the skills used in counselling is beyond the scope of this chapter and is covered in many other texts (Ivey et al 1987, Egan 1990, Burnard 1985, Nelson-Jones 1986). The main skills required, however, are identified in Fig.9.5. Effective helpers continually reflect on the counselling process, evaluate their use of these counselling skills and work towards constantly increasing their competence in applying them.

USING A FRAMEWORK

This chapter has suggested that counselling as a specific type of helping is grounded primarily in a way of being with others. Also, that competency in using interpersonal skills appropriately will enhance the effectiveness of the helper. The third side of the triangle (see Fig. 9.6) represents a model of helping. If a helper has access to a model and is able to apply it to these helping encounters then it is likely that the interactions will gain a sense of direction and clarity. A model is a framework which serves the helper by providing a map of the composite territory of counselling. Without this framework or map the complexity of the encounter may confuse or even overwhelm the helper and consequently the client is likely to feel lost too (see Fig. 9.7).

Models in nursing have a chequered history but this may be more to do with the way they have been applied than any shortcomings in the models themselves. A model is only of use to the extent that it serves clients' outcomes. It is not more important than the client and need not be rigidly adhered to in an inflexible manner. Models consist of sets of principles rather than magical formulae and if used wisely enable the helper to make sense of the process and provide direction (see Fig. 9.8).

Herink (1980) lists over 250 counselling and psychotherapeutic approaches, theories, schools, techniques and systems all claiming to lead to success. Since then many other new approaches have become established. To the novice helper this diversity of ideas may appear bewildering and even paralysing in terms of where to start.

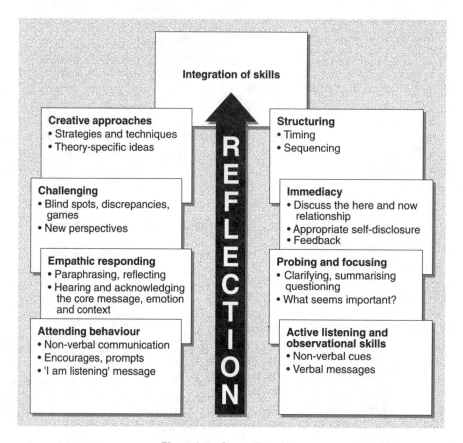

Integration of skills

Creative approaches
• Strategies and techniques
• Theory-specific ideas

Challenging
• Blind spots, discrepancies, games
• New perspectives

Empathic responding
• Paraphrasing, reflecting
• Hearing and acknowledging the core message, emotion and context

Attending behaviour
• Non-verbal communication
• Encourages, prompts
• 'I am listening' message

Structuring
• Timing
• Sequencing

Immediacy
• Discuss the here and now relationship
• Appropriate self-disclosure
• Feedback

Probing and focusing
• Clarifying, summarising questioning
• What seems important?

Active listening and observational skills
• Non-verbal cues
• Verbal messages

REFLECTION

Figure 9.5   Counselling skills

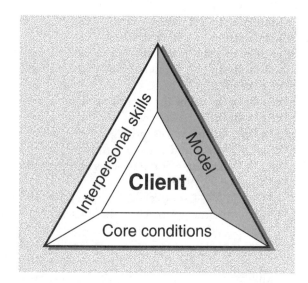

Figure 9.6   Using a framework for helping

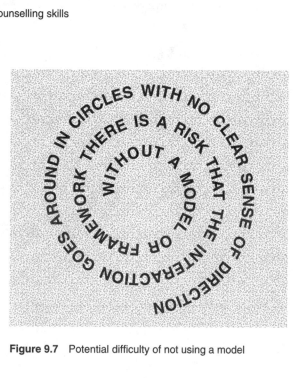

Figure 9.7   Potential difficulty of not using a model

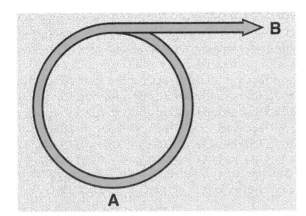

Figure 9.8   A model helps the client to reach a destination

An alternative way of thinking about these approaches is as a rich source of resources all containing points of merit and potential. Experienced counsellors, after gaining a thorough understanding of the various theories, are able to use ideas from these different approaches and integrate them into their own helping style.

Initially it is wise to learn and become competent with one practical working model or approach. Egan (1990) presents a model called the 'Skilled Helper' which he describes as a systematic approach to effective helping. It provides a pragmatic problem management approach that fits neatly within the process of nursing. It is described in some detail as one possible model which nurses may wish to explore further. The rich diversities of alternative models provide other options if the Skilled Helper does not suit.

The 'Skilled Helper'

This model of helping provides a practical way of working which is grounded in problem management and opportunity development. Egan (1990) claims the framework enables the helper to structure each step of the change process without ignoring the complexities. There is an emphasis on action that is grounded in the belief that the goal of helpers is to assist others to manage their lives more effectively. Another feature of the

skilled helper is that it is integrative in the sense that it enables helpers to use ideas and strategies from the wealth of different approaches within counselling and psychotherapy and to mould them into their own individual helping style.

The simplest and most logical way of describing this model is to progress in a linear fashion through the stages. This enables people to gain a conceptual understanding of the various steps. As helpers attain a behavioural understanding of the model and eventually a mastery of it they are able to use it much more flexibly by smoothly moving around within it. In other words, helping is not a linear process characterised by neat progressive steps; rather it is typically unpredictable and messy. This is why a map is essential to make sense of what is happening without losing the flexibility to respond to the uniqueness of each individual. The reader should bear these ideas in mind when considering the following stages in Figure 9.9.

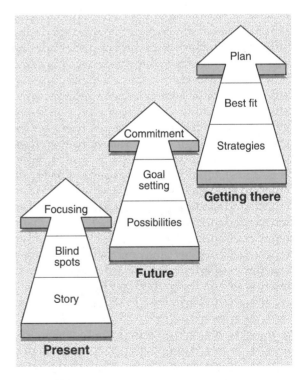

Figure 9.9   The Skilled Helper Model (adapted from Egan 1990).

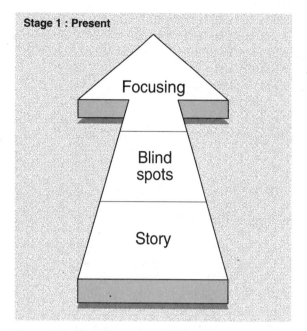

Stage 1 : Present

Figure 9.10 Stage 1: the present (adapted from Egan 1990).

Stage 1: the present

1.A: Telling the story. This stage involves the initial exploration and clarification of the situation, issues, problems and opportunities. As discussion progresses the helper is establishing a relationship with the client based on the essential core conditions and the helper's interpersonal skills. By listening to the story, the counsellor gains an understanding of what is going on for the client; through telling the story the client gains some clarity of her situation. A relationship is being established in which the client feels safe and is encouraged to disclose information.

1.B: Identifying and challenging blind spots. Egan (1990) suggests that most clients need to move beyond their initial subjective understanding of their problem situations. Limited perspectives of their situations may keep clients locked in self-defeating patterns of thinking and behaving. When faced with difficulties we tend to take a tunnel vision of our situations. Challenging blind spots does not consist of invalidating the client's experience or telling them what they are doing wrong. Effective challenging is grounded in empathy but allows the individual to examine alternative perspectives

or uncover information that they are selectively disregarding. Examples may include identifying hidden strengths and resources of the client or encouraging them to own their situation or problems. Challenging clients' perspectives is woven into the entire helping process, not just at this stage of the model.

When this challenging is done skilfully and with empathic sensitivity the client is prompted to examine her previously limited perspectives and see the difficulty in a different way. When done unskilfully with a lack of empathy the client is likely to feel criticised or misunderstood resulting in damage to the helping relationship.

1.C Focusing, screening and finding the leverage. Stage 1A explores the present situation. It provides an opportunity for the client to relate a broad and often complex jumble of events, feelings, thoughts and behaviours. In this format the story is rather unmanageable and so the helper now assists the client to filter out the major themes. This involves screening out the less significant parts of the story, focusing on the major issues and helping the client to decide which makes sense to work on first etc. Egan (1990) uses the word 'leverage' to mean the payoff for the client. For instance, the client may come to realise that working on one particular issue will, if managed successfully, contribute to the management of several other related problems. Stage 1C concentrates on breaking down the whole story into smaller, more manageable parts and helping the client to prioritise them.

Box 9.10 Challenging clients' perspectives
Alison is a student nurse who has recently failed her end of Common Foundation Programme examination. In addition to this a long-term relationship with a boyfriend has come to an emotional end. For some time things seem to have been going wrong in her life and during a tutorial she breaks down in tears. The tutor listens to Alison's story as she recounts her recent life. Alison blames herself for the fact that nothing has gone right for her. She sees nothing positive in her life and talks about herself in terms of a complete failure in relationships, studies and many other aspects of her life. While recognising and acknowledging the pain that Alison is feeling the tutor is able to sensitively point out areas of Alison's life that are successful and strengths and resources which she has demonstrated in her time at the college.

Stage 2 : Future

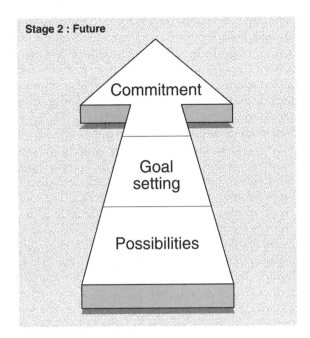

Figure 9.11 Stage 2: the future (adapted from Egan 1990).

Stage 2: the future

2.A: Possibilities. There comes a point when it is helpful to move the client on from talking about what is going wrong to what it is that they want. This stage is concerned with helping the client to look into the future. The question that moves people on is 'what would it look like if it were better?' This may seem an obvious question but it is one we rarely ask ourselves when we encounter a problem. More commonly, people find themselves in a problem situation and act before considering how they want things to be different. The fact that we tend not to ask this question of ourselves means that helpers often experience initial resistance at this stage. On the extreme level, a client who is depressed may see no future. If the helper can enable the client to construct the image of a possible future for themselves, she is doing something helpful. This stage also helps the process to move forward from what can become a self indulgent, excessive exploration of how awful the present is. Without such a step the process can go round in circles rather than moving towards outcomes.

Different techniques or strategies may be useful here. For clients who are resistive to this way of

---

Box. 9.11 What would it look like if it were better?

Lying in a hospital bed recovering from a recent operation provides time for Colin to think about his life. In particular he thinks about his relationship with his wife, Liz. He knows they have not been happy for some time and realises that they have both let this situation drift on.
One of the nurses spends some time listening to Colin and then asks 'what would your relationship with Liz be like if it was just how you wanted it?' This question takes Colin by surprise but after the nurse has left he finds himself thinking about the kind of relationship he would like to have with Liz. In many ways it is the relationship they used to have and he is able to see what is missing. He resolves to himself to work toward improving things in this way.

---

thinking, it may prove useful to encourage them to think how it would be if it were a *little* bit better. For others fantasy thinking may work e.g. if you could have whatever you want... If done sensitively this is not a tantalisation but a strategy to enable the client to realise what is within the dream that they value for themselves. The art of this stage lies in encouraging the client to free themselves from reality constraints or 'Ah, buts'. The use of creative strategies suited to the individual client is productive.

Box 9.12 What would it look like if it were a *little* better?

Steven has full-blown Aids. He sees a counsellor each week and has gradually come to experience these meetings as a safe haven in a world in which he feels unable to talk about what is happening to him. He has found it helpful to express his feelings and talk about his reaction to his changed circumstances. The focus of the interaction has been on the past and the circumstances that led to his situation today. At one of their meetings the counsellor asks Steven '*what is it that you want for yourself?*' This question stops Steven in his tracks and his initial response is rather abrupt '*I wouldn't have this wretched illness*'. The counsellor is able to help Steven to see past this angry response and gradually coaxes him to identify what things he does want for himself that would make a difference to his life. It emerges that he wants to patch up his relationship with some of his family; to increase his support network; to say the things he needs to say to others; to expand his social life. He is even able to talk about his own death and dying and how he would want that to be.

By asking the question in Box 9.12, the counsellor enabled Steven to rediscover his future. As often happens when people have a terminal illness, others avoid talking about the future. It is as if they have no future at all. By helping Steven to focus on possibilities in his life, the counsellor prompted him to realise what was really important to him and helped him to retrieve a sense of direction and future.

2.B: Goal setting. Once the possibilities have been generated by the client, it is timely to help them choose the ones that fit their circumstances. The broad pictures are forged into workable goals. The use of a behavioural checklist at this point may be helpful. Goals are more likely to be achieved if they are stated in terms of the checklist in Box 9.13.

2.C: Choice and commitment. Effective helpers leave the responsibility for choice with the clients. They can help the clients commit

themselves by helping them search for incentives for commitment. From the identified goals, which are the most urgent and immediate? Also the helper can enable the client to check out the costs and consequences of achieving the goals. For instance 'how much will achieving this goal cost me emotionally?' and 'what will be the effects on others in my life?'

If Stage 2 is done well the client will have a clear idea of what they would like to accomplish, without necessarily knowing how they will accomplish it.

Stage 3: Strategy—getting there

3.A: Strategies. A strategy is a set of actions designed to achieve a goal and tends to be more effective when chosen from a range of possibilities. If people attempt one strategy and fail they may assume that they will never achieve their goal, or they may try the same strategy again only to fail once more. Suggesting a range of ideas makes it more probable that one or a combination of them will suit the resources of the client. In this step the principle is to suspend judgement on the ideas (the 'ah, buts') and encourage the

Box 9.13	A behavioural checklist for goal setting
Accomplishment	What will be in place at the end of the day not *how* the client will get there i.e. stated in outcome terms.
Specific	Describe clearly and precisely what will be in place. Vague statements are unlikely to materialise into action.
Measurable	How will the client know when he/she has achieved the goal?
Realistic	Has the individual the resources to achieve the goal?
Owned	The goal must be the client's goal. He/she is not choosing it to please the counsellor or under pressure from third parties. It should be stated in 'I' terms.
Substantive	Achieving the goal should make a clear difference to the identified problem area.
Values	Is it within the client's values or will he/she find it too uncomfortable to achieve. How may it compromise the client's value system?
Time frame	Many of us live as if we are immortal. We will get round to it someday. Challenging the client to state a realistic and specific time frame for achieving the goal makes it more likely that it will be achieved.

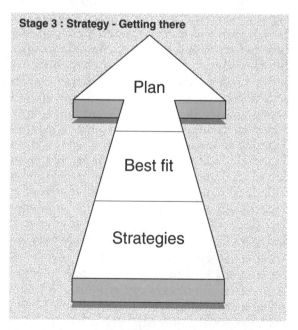

Figure 9.12 Stage 3: getting there (adapted from Egan 1990).

generation of as many different strategies as possible. One way of achieving this is to use brainstorming i.e. not to comment on each idea until after you have exhausted the possible list. Prompting the client to write them down ensures that none get lost in the process.

The helper uses prompts to encourage the client e.g. the people who may help, the places, the organisations etc. Often ideas piggyback on previous ideas and sometimes the use of humour or wild ideas is what is needed to get past the impasse to creativity.

Box 9.14 illustrates how generating a quantity of possible strategies Rose has increased her options. If she had not brainstormed the list with the Practice Nurse then she may have only tried the strategies that had not worked before. Rose probably would not use all of the strategies but would select the ones which best suited her.

3.B: Choosing the best strategies. The client, in collaboration with the helper, now reviews the different options and chooses the best single strategy or combination. The best strategy or combination of strategies are those which match the client's needs, preferences, resources and are least likely to be blocked by environmental

factors. In other words each strategy is reviewed to check whether it is realistic and within the client's values.

3.C: Turning strategies into plans. The chosen strategies need to be converted into a step-by-step plan which identifies the first task to be done, then the second etc., i.e. 'putting the flesh on the bones'. This planning should incorporate realistic time frames. The helper's intervention makes it more likely that the client will act and that she will receive support during that action. Remember that the plan is the client's plan, not the helper's. Throughout this model the helper's responsibility is for the process and the client's for the content and decisions. In this way the helper provides the conditions in which the client is able to face issues, make decisions and act on them.

Time spent identifying the possible factors which will either hinder or help the plan is worthwhile. Forewarned is forearmed and the inclusion of contingency plans will minimise the effect of hindering factors and maximise the effect of helpful factors.

The counselling relationship does not usually end here—the helper continues to meet the client to support her and to listen to her progress or lack of it.

An inexperienced helper, and sometimes even an experienced one, may apply the model too rigidly. It is worth stressing here once again that the model is at the service of client outcomes and needs to be managed with flexibility. A framework such as the Skilled Helper can make the process manageable rather than bewildering for the helper and the client.

PRACTICAL ISSUES

WHEN TO USE COUNSELLING

The art of effective helping is recognising the type of intervention that is required for a particular client in a given situation, taking into account their resources. Helping that is based on the values, skills and theories of counselling is only one part of the nurse's role. At other times

---

Box 9.14 Choosing a range of strategies

Rose desperately wants to give up smoking. Her health is deteriorating but all previous attempts to stop have failed. The practice nurse at the health centre offers to try and help. She asks Rose to write down all the possible ways she can think of to stop smoking. With encouragement Rose comes up with the following list:

- Join a support group for people trying to stop smoking.
- Tell everybody I know that I am going to stop.
- Try nicotine patches.
- Read books on the effects of smoking.
- Reward myself in some way for each day I don't smoke.
- Change my social patterns.
- Avoid places where others smoke.
- Spend the money I would spend on cigarettes on something else.
- Avoid shops that sell cigarettes.
- Start a keep fit routine to feel the benefits of a healthy lifestyle.
- Try hypnosis to stop.
- Meet with the practice nurse regularly for support.
- Discover things to eat that may replace the craving for cigarettes.

Box 9.15   Appropriate helping

David, a pre-registration Diploma student is on a short placement with a District Nurse. As he observes her working he is particularly impressed with her ability to adapt her interventions to match the needs and circumstances of the clients she visits. On one visit she recognises that a client requires advice and information regarding medication. This is given in a clear and unambiguous manner. The next visit requires a very different interaction as she uses counselling skills to enable a client to express his anguish at the recent death of his partner. David notices that both of these interventions are skilful and match exactly what the client requires.

---

the helping involves much more directive interactions such as advising, teaching, advocacy, prescribing etc.

So when is a counselling type of intervention appropriate? This is a difficult question to answer concisely and is as much involved with experience and sensitivity as with clear criteria. In assessing each situation the nurse recognises cues that provide the clues for deciding on the most appropriate type of helping.

The example in Box 9.15 demonstrates that the use of counselling skills is usually one part of the health carer's role. The art of helping is recognising clearly what is required based on sensitivity to the cues which the client provides.

SUPPORT AND SUPERVISION

This type of helping is complex and taxing for the helper. Helpers who take this route pay a price for doing so. The more effective helpers are at this work the more people will open up to them. This can contribute to an increased sense of burden and pressure. The effective helper identifies a clear network of people who provide support and knows how to access this support. Rather than a sign of weakness this represents a strength in the helper. Listening to what may often be painful experiences inevitably stimulates strong emotions in oneself. If these emotions are repressed then the helper is likely to pay the price in the long term. Off loading to trusted colleagues, co-counselling and support groups are all possible options for support.

Supervision is different to support. Practising counsellors require regular contact with an experienced counsellor who acts as a supervisor for their practice. Although most nurses are not counsellors, the more they use counselling skills in their work the greater the need for this type of supervision. Houston (1990) emphasises that a central task of the helper is to spend time to look again, in the presence of a supervisor, at what the helper and client said and did. The supervisor is primarily there to ensure that the client gets the best possible help from the counsellor. The benefits to the helper are supportive, developmental and educational through reflection on practice. The contracting of regular structured supervision is an important part of the counsellor's development. Fig. 9.13 illustrates the respective relationships of the three parties. The helper is the only person who is present in both the counselling and supervisory interactions and brings an account of the encounter with the client to the supervisor. Through discussion the counsellor gains a clearer and more objective perception of what may be happening in the counselling relationship.

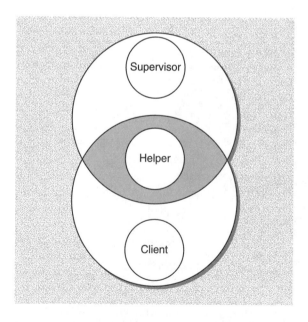

Figure 9.13 The supervision process (adapted from Hawkins & Shohet 1989)

Internal supervision

Casement (1985) argues that helpers need to develop their own capacity for spontaneous reflection within the session. He terms this reflection internal supervision. Over time helpers gradually shift from an initial dependence on their supervisors to a more independent internal supervision which is partly used to supplement external supervision. Developing an ability to process helping interventions at the same time as engaging in them is a requirement of the effective helper. Developing the ability to maintain an inner dialogue as an analysis of what is going on is an important part of the work. Paradoxically, one way of thinking about this activity of internal supervision is to externalise it by taking a helicopter view of the encounter. Imagine that you are on the ceiling looking down at yourself and the client; what do you observe? This perspective may be helpful in providing a sense of objectivity to the analysis.

The idea of internally monitoring what is going on at one level while concentrating so hard on what is being said, what you are saying, your use of skills, and where you are in the framework presents a complex picture. Surprisingly, as helpers develop their practice this seemingly impossible mixture of activities becomes more feasible. Box 9.16 suggests some reflective questions the helper may address when helping.

Reflecting on the process in this way both during and following the interaction represents a continuing challenge for the helper's self-development. Through reflection the helper is able to continually develop the ability to be more intentional in the way she works with others.

Box 9.16 Examples of internal supervision questions

1. How do I imagine the client is experiencing the relationship in the here and now?
2. How am I experiencing the relationship in the here and now?
3. What direction are we moving in?
4. What would be most helpful right now?
5. How much time do we have left and how does this affect what I do?
6. Am I concentrating or distracted—if so why?
7. Client's blind spots?
8. My blind spots?

SAFETY AND ETHICAL ISSUES

This type of helping is not neutral in terms of its effects and can be for better or worse (Egan 1990). Incompetent helpers can damage clients. Kagan (1973) questions whether all counsellors are competent and what happens if they are not. The first rule for the helper is to do no harm and this is achieved by maintaining the core conditions of the helping relationship and by contracting adequate supervision. An important aspect of the counselling relationship is for helpers to realise their limitations and know when it is appropriate to refer on to more specialist help.

TIME AND RESOURCES

A frequent comment from health carers is that they do not have the time to engage in this type of helping. In these days of economic restraint and limited resources the counselling relationship may be viewed as costly in terms of human resources. An alternative perspective is that time spent using counselling skills may actually be less demanding of resources in the long term. If the interaction results in a more accurate under-standing of the client's world, self-empowerment and independence, then this may be time profitably spent.

It is of mutual benefit to helper and client if the actual time available is openly negotiated at the outset. Whether this is ten minutes or one hour both parties then know when the interaction will end. This sets the boundary for the client to say what she wants to say and enables the helper to finish the interaction more easily. For those who engage in more formal counselling this time contracting is particularly important and usually includes negotiation of the number of sessions they will meet with the client.

CONCLUSION

This chapter has examined the nature of the counselling relationship in the context of health care, and the communication that takes place with it. Whilst recognising that most nurses and midwives are not counsellors they do provide psychological support to others as a part of their role. The principles of the counselling relationship have application for helpers in this capacity. The foundation of a helping relationship is based on core conditions or qualities, the most significant of these being the values of empathy, genuineness and respect.

Effective helping is also a skilled activity consisting of interpersonal or counselling skills which are underpinned by the core conditions. There are many different models or approaches within counselling and one function of these theories is to provide a sense of direction for the helper. The Skilled Helper is one example of a systematic problem management approach to effective helping.

Finally, it is suggested that reflection forms an integral part of the helper's development. Through the mechanisms of external and internal supervision helpers learn to ask questions of their practice, challenge their interventions and evaluate the quality of help they give to clients.

REFERENCES

Bond T 1989 Towards defining the role of counselling skills. Counselling, 69.3-9.

British Association of Counselling 1990 Code of ethics and practice for counsellors. BAC Office, Rugby.

Burnard P 1985 Learning human skills. Heinemann, London.

Burnard P, Morrison P 1991 Nurses' interpersonal skills. Nurse Education Today 11, pp.24-29.

Carkhuff R R 1970 Helping and human relations. Holt, Rinehart & Winston, New York.

Casement P 1985 On learning from the patient. Routledge, London.

Corey G 1986 Theory and practice of counselling and psychotherapy. Brooks/Cole, California.

Dryden W, Feltham C 1992 Brief counselling: a practical guide for beginning practitioners. Open University Press, Buckingham.

Egan G 1990 The skilled helper: a systematic approach to effective helping. Brooks/Cole, California.

Harre R 1980 Social being. Adams, New Jersey.

Harris C M 1987 Let's do away with counselling. In: Gray D (ed) The medical annual, pp. 105-111. Wright, Bristol.

Hawkins P, Shohet R 1989 Supervision in the helping professions. Open University Press, Buckingham.

Herink R 1980 The psychotherapy handbook: the A-Z guide to more than 250 therapies in use today. Meridian, New York.

Houston G 1990 Supervision and counselling. Rochester Foundation, London.

Howard A 1988 The necessities and absurdities of accredited helping. BAC Journal No. 64, July pp.19-22.

Ivey A E, Ivey M B, Simek-Downing L 1987 Counselling and psychotherapy: integrating skills theory and practice 2nd edn. Prentice-Hall, New Jersey.

Johnson W C, Heppner P P 1989 On reasoning and cognitive demands in counselling: implications for counsellor training. Journal of Counselling Development 67, pp. 428-429.

Kagan N 1973 Can technology help us toward reliability in influencing human interaction? Educational Technology 13, pp. 44-51.

Kalisch B J 1971 An experiment in the development of empathy in nursing students. Nursing Research May-June Vol. 20 No.3, pp. 202-211.

La Monica E, Carew D, Winder A, Hasse A, Blanchard K 1976 Empathy training as the major thrust of a staff development programme. Nursing Research 25, pp. 447-451.

Macleod Clark E 1985 The development of research in interpersonal skills in nursing. In: Kagan C (ed) Interpersonal skills in nursing: research and applications. Croom Helm, London.

Mearns D, Thorne B 1988 Person centred counselling in action. Sage, London.

Nelson-Jones R 1986 Human relationship skills. Cassell, London.

Patterson C H (ed) 1986 Theories of counselling and psychotherapy. 4th edn. Harper & Row, New York.

Pratt J 1990 The meaning of counselling skills. Counselling Journal Feb. pp.21-22.

Reynolds J 1987 Empathy: we know what we mean, but what do we teach? Nurse Education Today 7, pp.265-269 Longman Group, UK.

Rogers C 1951 Client centred therapy: its implications and theory. Houghton Mifflin, Boston.

Rogers C 1967 On becoming a person: a therapist's view of psychotherapy. Constable, London.

Stimson G, Webb B 1975 Going to see the doctor—the consultation process. In: General practice. Routledge & Kegan Paul, London.

Truax C, Mitchell K 1971 Research on certain therapist interpersonal skills in relation to process and outcome. In: Bergin A, Garfield S (eds) Handbook of psychotherapy and behaviour change. Wiley, New York.

Index